D1435598

THE RIGHT BITE

THE RIGHT BITE

Smart Food Choices for Eating on the Go

JACKIE LYNCH

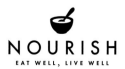

NOURISH
EAT WELL, LIVE WELL

In loving memory of my mother Terry,
an inspirational cook and a great believer
in the importance of good food.

The Right Bite
Jackie Lynch

First published in the UK and USA in 2016 by
Nourish, an imprint of Watkins Media Limited
19 Cecil Court
London WC2N 4EZ

enquiries@nourishbooks.com

Managing Editor: Rebecca Woods
Project Editor: Elinor Brett
Editor: Dawn Bates
Design Managers: Georgina Hewitt and
Viki Ottewill
Production: Uzma Taj

A CIP record for this book is available from
the British Library

ISBN: 978-1-84899-730-1

10 9 8 7 6 5 4 3 2 1

Typeset in Archer and Gravur Condensed
Colour reproduction by XY Digital
Printed in China

Publisher's note:
The information in this book is not intended
as a substitute for professional medical
advice and treatment. If you are pregnant or
are suffering from any medical conditions
or health problems, it is recommended that
you consult a medical professional before
following any of the advice or practice
suggested in this book. Watkins Media
Limited, or any other persons who have been
involved in working on this publication,
cannot accept responsibility for any injuries
or damage incurred as a result of following
the information contained in this book.

nourishbooks.com

CONTENTS

INTRODUCTION

The Right Bite is your solution to those difficult moments when you're faced with temptation and wondering what to eat or drink. Most of us have a fairly clear idea of what 'healthy eating' is all about, and it's not difficult to stick to a few key healthy principles when you're cooking at home and in control of the ingredients and the portion size. When you're out and about it's another story.

No one wants to be a party pooper, whatever the occasion – whether it's a quick coffee with friends, a celebration in a bar or a family picnic or barbecue. The challenge is how to join in and treat yourself without ruining the efforts that you make the rest of the time to keep things fairly healthy.

This is where *The Right Bite* can help by offering a specific solution to your dining dilemmas. Each chapter guides you through everyday social contexts, identifying the potential pitfalls of some choices and highlighting the advantages of others, making it both simple and clear how to identify *The Right Bite* in any given situation.

HOW TO USE THIS BOOK

Each of the chapters starts with an overview and then has features on individual foods. These features introduce the food, highlight the health pros and cons of that food, and include a series of information boxes. You can read all the features and become more informed quickly or you can save time by going straight to the food that's most relevant to you.

UNDERSTANDING KEY NUTRIENTS

This section offers a clear breakdown of how carbohydrate (including fibre, starch and sugar), protein and fats work in the body and explores current thinking on their impact on health. You might like to check back to this section, from time to time, to get some more detail on the nutrients discussed in each chapter.

CHAPTER OVERVIEW

At the start of each chapter there is a nutritional overview that draws out some of the key themes of the chapter, so you know what to expect. From there, the chapter contains a series of sections, made up of an introductory text to the food and different information boxes – The Right Bite, Nutrition Numbers and two fact boxes – to help you navigate your way through the material.

THE RIGHT BITE

If you're in a hurry, then just skip straight to this box in each food feature, as it offers a speedy solution. It will tell you all you need to know about the best thing to pick in that context, so that you can happily tuck into your muffin, cake, burger or other snack, confident in the knowledge that you're managing to limit the potential damage.

NUTRITION NUMBERS

For those who enjoy detail, there's plenty of opportunity to delve down into the nutritional information in the Nutrition Numbers box. This provides a breakdown of the principal and most relevant nutrients in the specific foods, displayed in grams, which allow for greater accuracy than imperial measurements. Where a nutrient is absent, it does not mean that it doesn't feature in the food, simply that the featured nutrients are either present in far greater quantity or are especially relevant to a particular health benefit or health risk. Where it refers to manufactured or pre-prepared foods, the values are based on an average from popular outlets or brands across a number of international regions, so that the information is as relevant as possible to you, wherever you're reading.

FASCINATING FACTS

Fact boxes are dotted throughout each chapter and aim to provide some extra nuggets of relevant and interesting information. Read them, store them away to share with friends or simply skip over them, as you choose.

UNDERSTANDING KEY NUTRIENTS

In this section, carbohydrate, fat and protein are all broken down into their component parts with an accessible explanation of each one, to help support the information that features in each chapter.

CARBOHYDRATE

WHAT IS CARBOHYDRATE?

Carbohydrate is the principal source of energy in most parts of the world where the human diet is built around cereal-based food, such as rice, bread or pasta, and starchy vegetables, such as potatoes. Carbohydrate is mostly derived from plant sources and is made up of sugar, starch and fibre.

WHAT ARE THE DIFFERENT TYPES OF CARBOHYDRATE?

Refined carbohydrate is when the nutritious whole grain of a plant has been stripped away, removing most of the fibre, along with any vitamins and minerals, leaving only the digestible starch and sugar. White bread, white rice and white pasta are everyday examples of refined carbohydrate. A simple carbohydrate is made up of only one or two units of sugar; they are very rapidly digested and provide a quick burst of energy. Typical sources include fruit, jams and honey. A complex carbohydrate is made up of a number of sugar molecules and they contain fibre, which makes them more satisfying. Vegetables, pulses and wholegrain foods are all sources of complex carbohydrate.

STARCH

Starch is made up of a number of glucose molecules and provides roughly the same level of energy as sugar, once it's been broken down by the body. It's important to take this into account when assessing the potential impact of a dish on your waistline and especially when you're reading a food label.

A typical carbohydrate section of a label may look like this:

```
Total carbohydrate      30g
Of which sugars         11g
Fibre                    2g
```

A simple calculation extracting the fibre and sugar leaves you with the total starch, which the body will quickly break down to the same level of energy as sugar:

$30g - 11g - 2g = 17g$ of starch

Adding the total starch and the total sugar together leaves you with 28g of digestible sugar in the body, the equivalent of 7 teaspoons of sugar.

$11g + 17g = 28g$ of digestible sugar

What Does Starch Do?

Starch has only one basic function, which is to convert into glucose in the body and provide a rapid source of fuel for the body's cells, powering the key bodily functions. The brain and the nervous system rely on glucose as the principal source of energy. As neurons cannot store glucose, the brain needs a steady supply for optimal function.

FIBRE

What is Fibre?

Fibre falls into three categories: indigestible non-starch polysaccharides (NSPs), resistant starch and lignin, which provides the woody structure to plant cell walls. When most people talk about fibre, they are referring to NSPs, which are made up of soluble and insoluble fibre.

NSPs are indigestible, so they pass straight into the bowel where they are fermented by the bacteria in the gut. The fermentation process increases levels of beneficial bacteria, promoting the formation of a healthy stool and helping to ensure optimal stool transit time.

Resistant starch passes through the intestine without being digested. Largely found in grains or potatoes, the proportion decreases with cooking but can increase when foods are cooled, so cold potatoes or cold pasta can contain fairly high levels of resistant starch, which may help to generate a sense of satiety.

What Does Fibre Do?

Fibre helps to slow down the release of glucose into the bloodstream, generating sustained energy levels, helping to regulate blood sugar levels and avoiding the spikes that lead to the release of insulin, a hormone that promotes the storage of excess sugar as fat cells. A fibre-rich diet keeps you going for longer and helps to limit cravings for sugary foods and carbohydrate, so it is helpful as part of a weight management programme.

The role of fibre in regulating digestive disorders such as constipation and diarrhoea is well documented, but the benefits go far beyond this. It helps to promote optimal levels of beneficial bacteria in the gut, and an increasing body of research suggests that this bacteria plays a vital role in health by modulating the gut immune system.

A fibre-rich diet rich helps to reduce the risk of chronic conditions such as bowel cancer, type 2 diabetes and cardiovascular disease. Soluble fibre (found in oats, apples and cruciferous vegetables, for example) is known to help with the regulation of cholesterol levels.

SUGAR

Too much sugar is the main culprit when it comes to weight gain and it has infiltrated the modern diet to a frightening extent. Sugar in all its different forms has a distinctly sweet taste, strong sensory appeal and can be highly addictive. Excessive intake of sugar is strongly associated with chronic conditions such as obesity, cardiovascular disease and type 2 diabetes.

Whatever form it is presented in, sugar is still sugar and, however you consume it, the impact on the body will be the same. The sugars that tend to feature most commonly as food additives are sucrose and fructose.

What Does Sucrose Do?

Sucrose is a natural plant sugar that is made up of one molecule of glucose and one of fructose. It is the benchmark of sugars by which the relative sweetness of sugar and artificial sweeteners are measured. Once ingested, sucrose is broken down into its component parts. Excessive levels of glucose can also be converted into triglycerides, which in large quantities are a risk factor for cardiovascular disease.

Regular consumption of high levels of sucrose can lead to a pre-diabetic condition known as insulin resistance, where the body cells become resistant to the action of insulin, allowing high levels of glucose to develop in the blood.

What Does Fructose Do?

Fructose is a single sugar molecule found in fruits; it's roughly three times as sweet as glucose and is increasingly used as an extract to sweeten soft drinks and desserts, in particular in the form of high fructose corn syrup. Extracting fructose from the fruit removes the all-important fibre element that is present when you eat the whole fruit and results in a very high dose of sugar. Whether this is done commercially by creating an additive or whether you're making your own juice, the impact will be the same.

The body processes fructose quite differently to glucose and it is largely metabolized by the liver, which brings a whole set of different problems when consumed to excess. There is growing evidence to suggest that high levels of processed fructose can contribute to non-alcoholic fatty liver disease and may increase the risk of developing type 2 diabetes.

What is Blood Sugar and How Does it Work?

The body is programmed to maintain steady levels of sugar in the blood, and too much or too little generates an emergency response to redress the balance. High glycaemic index (GI) foods in the form of sugar, refined and simple carbohydrates all lead to a spike in blood sugar and a consequent release of the hormone insulin, which encourages an initial storage of sugars in the liver and then stores any excess as fat. Once this process is complete, the blood sugar levels can drop significantly, generating the release of steroid (stress) hormones, cortisol and adrenaline, which create powerful cravings for sugary foods and refined carbohydrate. This may, in turn, lead to another blood sugar spike.

How Do Calories Work?

The unique way in which sugar is processed by the body has very real implications for people who aim to lose weight through a calorie-controlled diet. Essentially, all calories are not equal and the body will use them to perform different functions. This means that while a small 40g chocolate bar adds up to roughly the same calorie count as half an avocado or a small 40g portion of raw cashews, the body will deal with the calories from each food quite differently. The chocolate bar contains 20g of sugar, whereas the avocado contains 0.5g of sugar and the cashew only 2g. Of the three products, only the high-sugar chocolate bar is going to generate the insulin response and the subsequent storage of fat cells that leads directly to weight gain.

HOW MUCH CARBOHYDRATE SHOULD I EAT?

Current guidelines from the World Health Organization advise consuming at least 20g of fibre per day. Sugar guidelines are currently under consultation, with the general advice being that it should represent no more than 10% of daily calories consumed. In fact, the less sugar or refined carbohydrate in your diet, the better, as energy requirements can easily be fulfilled with an optimal diet of fibre and fat, which is an energy-rich nutrient.

FAT

WHAT IS FAT?

Fat is essential to the effective functioning of a range of bodily systems. It provides a rich source of energy, containing twice as much energy per gram as carbohydrate or protein. It is unfortunate that dietary fat shares a name with adipose tissue, otherwise known as fat cells, as this may have contributed to the popular misconception that dietary fat will make you fat. While excessive levels of certain types of fat may carry health risks, it is sugar and not fat that is the principal culprit in fat gain.

WHAT ARE THE DIFFERENT TYPES OF FAT?

Fats fall into four different categories: saturated fat, monounsaturated fats, polyunsaturated fats and trans fats. Fatty foods will always contain a blend of saturated, mono- and polyunsaturated fats – there is no food that contains only saturates or only polyunsaturates, for example, although the ratio between the fats can vary dramatically and one type will usually be dominant.

SATURATED FAT

Saturated fats are the simplest and most stable of the fats and can support cooking at high temperatures. They are mostly found in animal products, in particular red meat, dairy products and some vegetable sources, such as coconut oil.

Is Saturated Fat Bad For Me?

For a long time, saturated fat has been linked to increased risk of heart disease and strokes, which has resulted in a general move toward low-fat diets. However, it also plays a key part in some essential processes. Saturated fat promotes the production of cholesterol in the body and while the very word 'cholesterol' has become synonymous with heart disease and the risk of an early death, the human race would probably die out without cholesterol, as the body uses it to produce sex hormones such as testosterone and oestrogen. Other hormones, such as cortisol, which regulates the fight or flight response, and aldosterone, which supports fluid balance, are also produced using cholesterol. Without cholesterol we would be unable to manufacture vitamin D or bile acids, which are essential for optimal digestion. In short, while the jury may be out as to the role of excess cholesterol in heart disease, clearly some proportion of cholesterol is required for us to function at all.

The tide is currently turning with regard to the impact of saturated fat on health and on heart disease in particular. There is a school of thought that suggests that consuming saturated fat from natural sources, such as grass-fed beef, eggs and butter, may have direct health benefits, such as supporting the immune system, enhancing calcium absorption and strengthening cell membranes.

MONOUNSATURATED FATS

Monounsaturated fats are found in abundance in avocados, olive oil and nut oils, almonds, cashews, meat and whole milk products. Oils containing monounsaturates are typically liquid at room temperature and solid when chilled.

Are Monounsaturated Fats Good For Me?

Studies have shown that mono-unsaturated fats can help reduce levels of LDL cholesterol, which is considered to be the bad form of cholesterol. High levels of LDL are thought to be responsible for fatty deposits in the arteries, contributing to the risk of heart disease. However, the debate about the true impact of cholesterol and fat on heart health continues to rage on.

POLYUNSATURATED FATS

Polyunsaturates are the most complex and most interesting of the fats and are believed to have numerous health benefits. Their very complexity makes them more unstable, prone to oxidation and vulnerable to high temperature, which can generate harmful free radicals, increasing the risk of chronic disease. They fall into two principal categories known as omega 3 and omega 6.

Is Omega 3 Good For Me?

Omega 3 fatty acids are believed to lower the levels of harmful triglycerides, reduce blood clotting and decrease the risk of coronary heart disease. A diet rich in omega 3 can help to reduce inflammation, alleviating conditions such as rheumatoid arthritis, joint pain and asthma. There is also a possible association with the relief of symptoms of anxiety, low mood and depression. Omega 3 fatty acids are mostly found in oily fish, nuts and seeds and their associated oils.

Is Omega 6 Good For Me?

Omega 6 falls into two categories: linoleic acid and arachidonic acid. Principal sources of omega 6 are vegetable oils, such as palm or sunflower oil, and animal fats. High levels of vegetable oils are used in a range of processed and manufactured foods, such as cookies and cakes, as they prolong shelf life. This abundance of omega 6 is a double-edged sword: linoleic acid plays an important part in regulating hormones, relieving menstrual pain and reducing PMS symptoms, whereas excessive levels of arachidonic acid can result in swelling and inflammation and may contribute to chronic inflammatory conditions such as obesity and coronary heart disease. However, in correct doses, arachidonic acid supports cell function and brain and muscle development. Balancing the ratio of omega 6 to omega 3 is essential and current advice suggests that the omega

6:3 ratio should be anything from 1:1 to 5:1, rather than the current range of 20–50:1 prevalent in developed countries.

TRANS FATS

While the debate about saturated fat continues, health professionals are in no doubt about the danger of artificial trans fats. These are formed when fats are put through a hydrogenation process that hardens them and makes them solid at room temperature. This produces a butter substitute that is cheap and has a long shelf life, so that it is often used to produce a range of commercial baked goods.

The unnatural molecular form of these fats makes it difficult for the body to metabolize them as it would other fats and this means that trans fats tend to remain in the circulation, resulting in cellular damage and significantly increasing the risk of cardiovascular disease and some cancers.

Levels of artificial trans fats in food products are legislated and food manufacturers are starting to use lower levels now that the health risks have become apparent. However, any food label that contains the words 'partially hydrogenated fats' indicates that the product contains trans fats.

THE LOW-FAT TRAP

As all foods that contain fat are made up of saturated, mono- and polyunsaturated fats, there is a real risk of throwing the baby out with the bath water, as manufacturers don't carefully distinguish between which fat to extract from a food. As the fat is stripped out, so is much of the flavour, so that it's common for low-fat products to contain high levels of added sugar or salt to compensate.

HOW MUCH FAT SHOULD I EAT?

Current guidelines recommend consuming around 70g of fat per day, broken down into 20g of saturated fat per day for women and 30g for men, leaving the remainder to be made up of mono- and polyunsaturates. While health professionals continue to debate the exact impact of saturated fats on heart health, it would be advisable to remain within these limits and to focus on quality sources, such as fresh meat, eggs and cheese, rather than deep-fried processed products. Foods that contain high levels of omega 3, such as flaxseed, may need to be used in moderation by people who have been prescribed anticoagulant medication, due to its blood-thinning properties.

PROTEIN

WHAT IS PROTEIN?

The human body is largely composed of protein and, along with water, it makes up the greatest proportion of our body weight. It is vital for cell function and the growth and repair of bones, organs, glands, muscles, ligaments, tendons, skin, hair and nails. It underpins the overall development of the human body as it forms the basis of chromosomes and the genetic code in cell DNA is used to make proteins. Protein is also responsible for regulating a range of processes in the body as it makes up the hormones and enzymes that oversee so many bodily functions. Proteins help to regulate the body's fluid balance and play a part in ensuring the exchange of nutrients between tissue, blood, lymph and intercellular fluids.

In other words, we can't function without protein.

WHAT ARE THE DIFFERENT TYPES OF PROTEIN?

Protein is made up of building blocks called amino acids and each type of protein requires a different composition of amino acids in a unique sequence in order to carry out a specific role in the body. There are 22 standard amino acids required to cover our bodily functions but only nine are known as 'essential amino acids', which need to be acquired through the diet. The body then combines these amino acids to develop the remaining 13.

ARE ALL PROTEIN FOODS THE SAME?

Animal proteins such as meat, fish and eggs contain all the essential amino acids in one easy package, but vegetarians and vegans may have to work a little harder, as plant sources of proteins generally contain some but not all the required amino acids, which is why a diet with a broad variety of plant protein is so important. There are some notable exceptions, such as quinoa, hemp seed, soy bean and amaranth, which contain all the essential amino acids

WHAT IS THE FUNCTION OF ESSENTIAL AMINO ACIDS?

Essential amino acids perform a very wide range of different functions and fall into different groupings. Isoleucine, leucine and valine are branched-chain amino acids, so called because of their molecular structure. These play a key role in bone, muscle and tissue repair, as well as promoting energy production and increasing endurance. They are much in demand among athletes and exercise enthusiasts, but it's worth bearing in mind that they will also have a very positive effect for anyone looking to recover from injury or surgery, for example.

Tryptophan and phenylalanine support neurotransmitter function in the brain, helping to regulate mood, manage pain and support memory and learning, as well as underpinning the function of the central nervous system.

Histidine and methionine have a detoxifying effect and help to neutralize the impact of pollutant heavy metals such as mercury, lead and cadmium. Threonine and lysine are required for antibody production and the formation of collagen, a key component of skin, hair and nails.

HOW MUCH PROTEIN SHOULD I EAT?

While protein is an essential nutrient and should form part of a balanced diet, excessive levels of protein will not enhance its many functions but simply place an extra burden on the liver and kidneys by allowing harmful toxins to build up.

Current advice suggests that protein should form roughly 20% of overall nutrient intake per day, although requirements may vary considerably, depending on age, growth requirements, levels of exercise and state of health. A simple guideline would be to ensure that protein-rich food represents roughly a quarter of the overall meal at lunch and dinner, and that it is present in some form at breakfast and snacks.

Breakfast on the Go

saving your bacon

Breakfast is full of pitfalls for the unwary, and the combination of feeling sleepy and being short of time is really not conducive to making smart food choices. It's important to get it right, because it's an essential meal, as your body needs fuel to start the day effectively. Blood sugar is low in the morning, resulting in high levels of the stress hormone, cortisol. Excessive cortisol encourages the breakdown of muscle instead of fat, a key consideration if you work out before breakfast.

It's easy to assume that by skipping breakfast you can help weight loss by reducing calories. Actually, the reverse is true, as it generates a hormonal response that has a direct impact on your waistline. Ghrelin is the hormone that manages appetite and it increases before a meal and decreases after a meal. Studies have shown that people who miss breakfast eat more at lunch and dinner than people who regularly eat breakfast, because ghrelin levels remain unchecked.

> Skipping breakfast generates a hormonal response that has a direct impact on your waistline

The best breakfast is a blend of protein and fibre, which maintains blood sugar levels and ensures sustained energy, helping to avoid the mid-morning munchies. Unfortunately, it's easy to fall into the habit of having dessert for breakfast, as a lot of quick and easy options when you grab breakfast on the run tend to be full of sugar.

Your body will burn through a high-sugar breakfast quickly, leading first to a blood sugar spike, encouraging your body to store any excess sugar as fat, and then to a blood sugar crash, resulting in powerful sugar cravings and poor food choices. This can greatly affect energy levels, concentration and physical performance.

Smart forward planning is of real benefit here: checking out the online menu of your favourite outlet and identifying the best option in advance can save you precious time and your waistline from unwanted extra inches.

CROISSANTS

A delicious, light, flaky croissant may seem the obvious and irresistible accompaniment to your morning coffee but there's little in the way of good news on the health front. That unique flaky effect is created by using a technique involving a large quantity of butter, similar to making puff pastry, and even if you choose a basic, unflavoured croissant, you'll be consuming half the guideline daily amount of saturated fat before you even get to work.

The other key component of croissants is refined carbohydrate, which can be as much as 45g per croissant, depending on your choice, roughly the equivalent of 3 average slices of white bread, and the fast route to a blood sugar spike before you even start to take the

BUTTER IS PARTICULARLY RICH in butyric acid, a short-chain saturated fatty acid, which helps to feed the friendly bacteria that are important for optimum digestion in the gut.

NUTRITION NUMBERS
per unit

↳ PLAIN CROISSANT
Calories: 309 » Carbohydrate: 31g
Sugars: 4g » Saturated fat: 12g
Protein: 6g

↳ ALMOND CROISSANT
Calories: 423 » Carbohydrate: 45g
Sugars: 18g » Saturated fat: 11g
Protein: 8g

↳ HAM & CHEESE CROISSANT
Calories: 353 » Carbohydrate: 23g
Sugars: 4g » Saturated fat: 10g
Protein: 16g

↳ PAIN AU CHOCOLAT/ CHOCOLATE CROISSANT
Calories: 318 » Carbohydrate: 29g
Sugars: 9g » Saturated fat: 10g
Protein: 5g

added sugar into account. While the almond croissant may seem a deceptively healthier choice, it actually comes out top in terms of sugar content, containing nearly 5 teaspoons of added sugar, so this is definitely one to watch if weight management is important to you. You may think there's an advantage to be had from the vitamin and mineral content of almonds, but as studies have shown that the skin is the most nutrient-rich part of the nut and the recipe calls for blanched almonds, the disadvantages of this croissant far outweigh the potential benefits. It will, of course, come as no surprise to learn that a pain au chocolat or chocolate croissant also scores pretty high on the sugar scale, almost double the sugar content of a plain croissant.

The savoury options, such as ham and cheese croissants, are a possibility worth considering, as the sugar content is lower and they contain more than twice the amount of protein than the sweet versions, making them a more satisfying option for breakfast. However, if heart health or cholesterol levels are a concern for you, then you may prefer to enjoy these sparingly, due to the

THE RIGHT BITE

A croissant is never going to be the smartest breakfast option, so it's best to keep it as a very occasional treat. You could limit the damage by opting for a savoury croissant, as this will help to keep the sugar content down and contains some protein, which will help to keep you going. Otherwise, a basic plain croissant is the one to choose, as long as you don't make the mistake of adding a helping of honey or jam, which really won't help matters.

high level of salt (almost half the daily recommended limit) and the saturated fat in the added cheese and ham.

CHEWING, ABSORBING AND PROCESSING FOOD all burns energy (up to 200 calories per day). This is called the thermic effect of food. Processing protein uses more energy than other foods, which is another reason why a protein-rich breakfast is a smart move.

TOAST

If your taste runs to grabbing a quick slice of toast on the run, this isn't automatically an unhealthy option, but much will depend on your choice of bread. The higher the level of fibre, the more satisfying your toast will be, generating sustained energy that will keep you going for longer. This means that it's always better to choose a form of wholegrain bread – even a basic wholemeal loaf contains twice the amount of fibre of white bread, and both granary and rye bread contain even more fibre.

A high-fibre option won't just help to maintain blood sugar levels, it will also help to contribute to a healthy digestion. Fibre plays an important part in the formation and passage of healthy stools. Soluble fibre found in rye bread can help to soften stools and relieve constipation

BURNT TOAST GENERATES a chemical called acrylamide, which has been associated with increased risk of some cancers, so it's best to opt for lightly toasted bread.

NUTRITION NUMBERS
per 40g slice

↳ WHITE TOAST
Calories: 87 » Carbohydrate: 18g
Sugars: 1g » Fibre: 0.7g
Magnesium: 11mg

↳ WHOLEMEAL TOAST
Calories: 87 » Carbohydrate: 17g
Sugars: 1g » Fibre: 2g
Magnesium: 30mg

↳ GRANARY (SEEDED) TOAST
Calories: 108 » Carbohydrate: 17g
Sugars: 1g » Fibre: 3g
Magnesium: 32mg

↳ RYE TOAST
Calories: 76 » Carbohydrate: 19g
Sugars: 0.2g » Fibre: 4g
Magnesium: 34mg

and insoluble fibre in wholemeal bread helps to move the stool through the gut.

If you struggle with IBS-like symptoms such as bloating, flatulence or inconsistent bowel movements, then you might prefer to opt for 100% rye bread rather than wheat bread. Wheat can be an irritant to a sensitive gut, especially at times of stress, and may exacerbate these symptoms.

Another potential health benefit of choosing wholegrain breads is the mineral content, as whole grains are a very good source of magnesium, which supports the nervous system, as well as regulating muscle action. A deficiency in magnesium is commonly associated with muscle twitches or cramps, such as calf cramps or eyelid twitches.

If you opt for granary bread, then you could be gaining some other residual health benefits, as the seeds in a granary loaf are rich in poly- and monounsaturated essential fatty acids that contribute to heart health, as well as helping to ease inflammatory conditions such as joint pain or eczema.

Finally, don't neglect to choose your topping with care. A protein source

THE RIGHT BITE

The best all-round option here would be 100% rye toast as it's the highest in fibre, the lowest in sugar and contains marginally more magnesium than the other wholegrain offerings. It also has the advantage of being far kinder to the digestion than wheat-based breads. Match it with a protein topping and you're good to go.

is the perfect accompaniment to your toast, to maintain blood sugar balance and keep you going throughout the morning. Sugar-free peanut butter or cottage cheese will always be a much more sustaining choice than honey, jam or yeast extract.

COOKING FOOD AT HIGH TEMPERATURES generally reduces magnesium content by approximately 20%. However, in the case of toast there is actually a marginal increase in magnesium levels, so that you can still enjoy the health benefits.

EGG & BACON ROLL

Eggs have had a bad press for a long time because they contain cholesterol. However, repeated studies have shown that dietary cholesterol does not lead to the high levels of bad cholesterol in the blood that are currently believed to be associated with heart disease.

Eggs are highly nutritious and an excellent source of lean protein, making them an ideal breakfast food. Don't make the mistake of eating just the egg

THE BEST SOURCE OF VITAMIN D is through exposure to sunlight, but egg yolk is one of the few foods that contains a small amount of dietary vitamin D. Optimum vitamin D levels have long been associated with healthy bones and teeth and there is now some research to suggest that it may also play a broader role in health that includes supporting the immune system and mental health.

NUTRITION NUMBERS
per unit

↳ GRILLED BACON (per 2 slices)
Calories: 140 » Protein: 12g
Total fat: 11g » Saturated fat: 4g
Salt: 3g

↳ FRIED EGG
Calories: 100 » Protein: 7g
Total fat: 8g » Saturated fat: 1.5g
Salt: 0.4g

↳ EGG & BACON ROLL
(white bread)
Calories: 407 » Protein: 27g
Carbohydrate: 30g » Sugars: 3g
Fibre: 2g » Total fat: 22g
Saturated fat: 6g » Salt: 4g

↳ EGG & BACON ROLL
(wholemeal bread)
Calories: 425 » Protein: 27g
Carbohydrate: 29g » Sugars: 2g
Fibre: 4g » Total fat: 21g
Saturated fat: 6g » Salt: 4g

white as the yolk is the most nutritious part, full of antioxidants such as zinc, selenium and vitamin E, as well as being a great source of iron and healthy monounsaturated fats believed to promote heart health. Yolk also contains iodine, which plays a key role in healthy thyroid function.

If you need to monitor saturated fat levels, a poached or hard-boiled egg in the roll instead of a fried egg will significantly reduce the fat content.

The news is not so good when it comes to bacon, as it's a highly processed meat that comes with a number of health concerns. Just 2 slices take up half the recommended daily limit of salt in the diet, so bacon is one to avoid if high blood pressure is a concern. Cured meats contain chemical preservatives such as nitrates and nitrites and while levels of these are carefully regulated, there remains a potential association with an increased risk of gastrointestinal cancers. This suggests that bacon should be enjoyed as an occasional treat.

Choosing a wholemeal roll will ensure optimum levels of complex carbohydrate, which will keep you going

THE RIGHT BITE

The smart move here is to keep it simple and leave out the bacon, opting for a wholemeal egg roll. This way you dramatically reduce the levels of salt and preservatives. As well as ensuring you enjoy all the residual health benefits of the egg, it provides the ideal breakfast blend of protein and fibre and this will help to keep you going throughout the morning.

for longer throughout the morning. It's also best to be cautious when it comes to the potential added extras – a generous serving of ketchup adds the equivalent of 2 teaspoons of sugar and melted cheese can add a hefty dose of saturated fat.

IF IT'S THE MORNING AFTER THE NIGHT BEFORE then an egg could be just the thing to perk you up. Eggs are rich in the amino acid cysteine, which has antioxidant properties that help break down toxins in the liver.

BAGELS

There's a lot more to a bagel than a bread roll with a hole in the middle, although many of the commercial offerings boil down to just that. The traditional chewy texture of a good bagel is due to the strong bread flour, which is rich in protein, promoting the formation of higher levels of gluten in the dough. Bagels are made with a generous helping of sugar or malt syrup, giving them the characteristic shiny tinted crust and making them sweeter than the average bread roll.

When it comes to choosing the healthy options for bagels, the same rules apply as with bread – the high-fibre options are the ones that tick all the boxes. A multi-seed or wholemeal bagel contains twice as much fibre as

PEANUT BUTTER IS A GREAT SOURCE of plant protein, as well as being full of essential mono- and polyunsaturated fats, so it could be a really healthy topping for your bagel, as long as you steer clear of the brands with added sugar.

NUTRITION NUMBERS
per unit

↳ PLAIN BAGEL
Calories: 230 » Carbohydrate: 44g
Sugars: 4g » Fibre: 3g » Salt: 0.7g

↳ CINNAMON & RAISIN BAGEL
Calories: 263 » Carbohydrate: 50g
Sugars: 8g » Fibre: 3g » Salt: 0.8g

↳ SEEDED BAGEL
Calories: 266 » Carbohydrate: 47g
Sugars: 5g » Fibre: 5g » Salt: 0.8g

↳ MULTIGRAIN BAGEL
Calories: 295 » Carbohydrate: 58g
Sugars: 5g » Fibre: 6g » Salt: 1g

↳ WHOLEMEAL BAGEL
Calories: 248 » Carbohydrate: 41g
Sugars: 5g » Fibre: 7g » Salt: 1g

the plain or sweetened versions and this slow-release carbohydrate will set you up for sustained energy throughout the morning. Opting for a wholegrain version has the added benefit of supporting optimal digestion, as whole grains are rich in fibre, which is essential for the formation and easy passage of stools. They're also an excellent source of magnesium, which is required for peristalsis, the muscle contraction that moves the stool through the bowel and helps to keep things 'regular'.

Watch out for sweetened bagels that contain dried fruits as they don't have much to offer in the way of nutrients – just a mix of sugar and refined carbohydrate, both of which will add inches to your waistline if you eat them regularly. They're also unlikely to satisfy you for any length of time, leaving you open to the temptation of a sugary mid-morning snack.

If you want to make the most of your bagel, then a careful choice of topping could make all the difference, turning this into a really quality breakfast option. Try to avoid the obviously sugary options of jam or chocolate spread.

THE RIGHT BITE

You could do a lot worse than opt for the classic smoked salmon and cream cheese option with cracked black pepper and a wholegrain bagel. This is a deliciously winning combination of protein and fibre that ticks the blood sugar box and will keep you on the straight and narrow all morning. Hidden extra benefits include the polyunsaturated fats in the salmon, a brain boosting start to the day, and piperine in the black pepper, a compound that helps to promote nutrient absorption in the intestine.

ALTHOUGH YEAST EXTRACT CONTAINS virtually no macronutrients, it is heavily fortified with B vitamins, which play a key part in energy production and the function of the nervous system. This is an extra bonus for vegans, as vitamin B12 is found almost exclusively in animal products and a plant-based diet can lead to a deficiency, otherwise known as pernicious anaemia.

PORRIDGE

If your instinct is to grab a porridge/oatmeal pot on the way in to work, then you're already halfway to an excellent start to the day. Traditional porridge consists of oats cooked with water or milk and a dash of salt. It's an excellent source of soluble fibre, which plays a key role in helping to regulate cholesterol levels. In fact, studies have shown that ensuring a minimum of 9g of soluble fibre in the form of oats each day can help to reduce levels of bad LDL cholesterol.

Starting the day with porridge is also a great option if weight management is your goal, as it helps to maintain a blood sugar balance right at the start of the day. Porridge is low in sugar and high in complex carbohydrate, which will ensure sustained energy levels that keep you

VEGETARIANS NEED TO BE AWARE that oats contain high levels of phytates that can inhibit the absorption of non-heme (plant) sources of iron and may result in a deficiency.

NUTRITION NUMBERS
per 300g (cooked weight)

↳ PORRIDGE/OATMEAL
Calories: 235 » Carbohydrate: 31g
Sugars: 9g » Protein: 11g
Fibre: 4g

TOPPINGS
per 35g serving

↳ FRUIT COMPOTE
Calories: 36 » Sugars: 5g
Protein: 0.2g

↳ HONEY
Calories: 108 » Sugars: 26g
Protein: 0.1g

↳ CHOPPED BANANA
Calories: 28 » Sugars: 6g
Protein: 0.4g

↳ SUNFLOWER SEEDS
(10g tablespoon)
Calories: 57 » Sugars: 0.1g
Protein: 2g

going for longer, helping you to avoid the temptation of a sugary mid-morning snack.

There's a surprisingly good level of protein in oats, which helps contribute to the protein-fibre balance that's so important for a healthy and satisfying breakfast, although adding seeds or nuts will provide a perfect boost of protein, fibre and omega 3 in one easy package. Pumpkin seeds, sunflower seeds or chopped walnuts are all simple additions that will support the overall health profile of the dish, and a topping of fresh fruit, such as blueberries, adds a natural sweetness along with lots of antioxidants.

The pitfalls with porridge come with the toppings – if you're picking it up from your favourite outlet en route to work, then it's easy to be tempted by one of the sugary toppings on offer. A small 35g topping of honey adds the equivalent of 6 teaspoons of sugar to the dish, undoing a lot of the good work of choosing porridge in the first place. You also need to be wary of the quick and easy microwaveable sachets of flavoured porridge, as these contain a minimum of 2 teaspoons of sugar.

THE RIGHT BITE

The best possible option is plain porridge with milk or natural yogurt, with a dash of cinnamon or some fresh berries. If there isn't the option to add seeds on the spot, then keep a stash of raw pumpkin or sunflower seeds in your desk and add a large spoon when you get to work.

One smart way to perk up the flavour of your porridge without doing any damage is to add a dash of cinnamon to it instead. This can help to maintain blood sugar balance as some studies have shown that cinnamon helps to regulate blood glucose levels.

OATS ARE A RICH SOURCE OF BETA GLUCANS, compounds that can modulate the gut immune system by activating and enhancing the action of immune cells, helping to avoid niggling and lingering colds and infections through the winter months.

GRANOLA & MUESLI POTS

A granola or muesli pot may seem like the natural choice if you're trying to keep things healthy, as a blend of raw or cooked oats, fresh or dried fruit and a few nuts sounds like a winning combination. The problem is that the handy little pots that are available in so many breakfast outlets come with a number of hidden traps that mean that they may not be as healthy as you imagine.

The problem is that many of these products really do go overboard on the sugar content, which can feature in a variety of different ways. The first thing to look for is just how much there is in the way of dried fruit in your favourite breakfast pot. The drying process

> **THE DRYING PROCESS** can destroy the vitamin C content of fruit as well as drastically increasing the sugar content, so fresh fruit is always going to be a healthier option in your granola or muesli pot.

↳ GRANOLA FRUIT POT
Calories: 359 » Carbohydrate: 42g
Sugars: 23g » Protein: 6g
Fibre: 4g

↳ BIRCHER MUESLI
Calories: 305 » Carbohydrate: 51g
Sugars: 33g » Protein: 8g
Fibre: 4g

TOPPINGS
per 10g tablespoon

↳ SUNFLOWER SEEDS
Calories: 57 » Sugars: 0.1g
Protein: 2g » Polyunsaturates: 3g

↳ PUMPKIN SEEDS
Calories: 56 » Sugars: 0.1g
Protein: 3g » Polyunsaturates: 2g

↳ FLAXSEEDS
Calories: 57 » Sugars: 0.1g
Protein: 2g » Polyunsaturates: 3g

concentrates the fruit sugar considerably, so it's a far more sugary option than the original fresh fruit. Then there's the fruit puree, which is a common addition to the pot and fruit sugar is still sugar, even if it's in a more natural form than refined sugar. There's also the binding to take into consideration: with granola the oats are commonly bound with a blend of honey or syrup and oil before they're baked and with bircher muesli, the oats are usually soaked in apple juice overnight. Honey and fruit juice are just sugar in another guise. When you add all of this up, it's no surprise that the average muesli or granola pot can contain the equivalent of 6–8 teaspoons of sugar, which is always going to be an issue if you're watching your weight.

On the plus side, oats and dried fruit are excellent sources of soluble fibre, which encourages regular bowel movements by moving waste matter through the gut, so they are a good option for anyone with a sluggish digestion. Oats also contain compounds that can help to regulate cholesterol levels, and as a complex carbohydrate they will help to slow down the sugar release into

THE RIGHT BITE

Based on the numbers, there isn't a great deal to choose between the two, but the muesli has a slight edge as raw oats and raw apple retain more nutrients than cooked oats and fruit puree. Either way, the trick is to keep the sugar to a minimum, so try to limit the sugars by opting for a pot with dried fruit or fruit puree but not both. You might want to try adding a tablespoon of sunflower, pumpkin and ground flaxseed as this will provide protein, fibre and omega 3 in one easy hit, seriously boosting the health benefits of your breakfast.

the bloodstream, keeping you going for longer than the refined carbohydrate found in many commercial cereals.

RAISINS ARE ACTUALLY DRIED GRAPES but there's a world of difference in the sugar content, as they contain roughly four times as much sugar as grapes.

YOGURT

In its basic form, yogurt has much to recommend it, and the easy availability of a single-serving yogurt pot makes it a practical option for breakfast on the run. Despite the plethora of low-fat products that are available, whole milk yogurts are not excessively high in fat and by skimming off the fat, much of the flavour is lost, so the manufacturers tend to add in extra sugar and artificial sweeteners to boost the flavour.

There is a persistent assumption that eating low-fat yogurt is the best option for a healthy diet. In fact this is not the case. Full-fat yogurt contains a very small amount of saturated and monounsaturated fats, hardly enough to be of any concern and certainly not worth the large amounts of sugar that feature

SOME PEOPLE WHO ARE LACTOSE INTOLERANT find that yogurt doesn't cause the same digestive problems as milk as the yogurt-making process has converted the lactose into lactic acid.

NUTRITION NUMBERS
per 150g pot

↳ LOW-FAT FRUIT YOGURT
Calories: 117 » Sugars: 20g
Fat: 2g » Protein: 6g

↳ FULL-FAT FRUIT YOGURT
Calories: 163 » Sugars: 24g
Fat: 4g » Protein: 6g

↳ NATURAL LOW-FAT YOGURT
Calories: 59 » Sugars: 8g
Fat: 0g » Protein: 6g

↳ NATURAL FULL-FAT YOGURT
Calories: 82 » Sugars: 6g
Fat: 4g » Protein: 6g

↳ LOW-FAT GREEK YOGURT
Calories: 86 » Sugars: 7g
Fat: 0g » Protein: 7g

↳ FULL-FAT GREEK YOGURT
Calories: 186 » Sugars: 7g
Fat: 6g » Protein: 6g

as a replacement in low-fat offerings. It is also worth noting that saturated fat is not something to avoid at all cost, as it plays an important role in a number of areas, such as the production of sex hormones.

The word 'yogurt' has become synonymous with 'health', but there is a vast difference between natural yogurt, fruit yogurt and flavoured yogurt. Fruit and flavoured yogurts whether low-fat or full-fat can contain the equivalent of up to 6 teaspoons of sugar, which is more than the average chocolate chip cookie you'd find in a coffee bar.

One of the major health benefits of yogurt is that it is a source of the beneficial bacteria that is so important for optimum health. The gut is made up of billions of these strains of bacteria that play a key part in regulating digestive health and modulating the immune system. All unpasteurized yogurts contain beneficial bacteria, not just the ones that market themselves as having 'probiotic' properties. If you want to derive optimum benefit from these beneficial bacteria, avoid sugary yogurts or yogurt drinks, as they contain high levels of sugar, which feed the unfriendly

THE RIGHT BITE

With yogurt, the healthy option is very clear cut: the best choice is a natural full-fat yogurt (with full-fat Greek yogurt as a close second), as this is lowest in sugar. It avoids all the additives and preservatives that feature in flavoured and fruit yogurts, so that you can enjoy all the natural health benefits of the product. If you need to add a little sweetness, try adding chopped apple or blueberries as these are far higher in fibre and antioxidants than fruit puree.

bacteria in the gut, and this may result in an imbalance of gut bacteria resulting in symptoms of bloating and wind.

AS WELL AS BEING A SOURCE OF CALCIUM, yogurt is one of the few foods to contain small amounts of vitamin D. As vitamin D helps to promote calcium absorption, yogurt could be a good option if bone health is a consideration.

JUICES

Juicing can be a quick and easy way to ensure a fast blast of vitamins, minerals and antioxidants. It's easy to feel a certain satisfaction in grabbing a quick juice in the morning and ticking off one or two of the recommended five-a-day of fruit and vegetables. However, many juices can be high in sugar and little else, which rather defeats the object if you're trying to be healthy.

Freshly squeezed juice oxidizes very quickly when it's exposed to oxygen, which is why it can taste a little strange if you leave it for a while before drinking it. Yet fresh, cartoned juices have a fridge life of around 3 days. The pasteurization process intensifies the natural fruit

LEAFY GREEN VEGETABLES are a powerhouse of vitamins and minerals, containing more than twice as much vitamin C as an orange, as well as being an excellent source of energy-boosting iron and B vitamins, calming magnesium and bone-building calcium.

NUTRITION NUMBERS
per 250ml serving

↳ ORANGE JUICE
Calories: 90 » Sugars: 22g
Fibre: 0.5g

↳ CARROT JUICE
Calories: 50 » Sugars: 9g
Fibre: 1.5g

↳ GREEN JUICE (with kale, cucumber, parsley, 1 apple)
Calories: 101 » Sugars: 12g
Fibre: 2g

↳ TOMATO JUICE
Calories: 35 » Sugars: 7g
Fibre: 1g

sugars and, as a preservative, sugar gives the product a longer shelf life. So when you're happily quaffing a large glass of orange juice you're also consuming the equivalent of almost 6 teaspoons of sugar.

If you're able to have freshly squeezed juice, then this will help to circumvent part of the problem, but one of the challenges of fresh juicing is that most of the fibre is left in the waste section of the machine. If you're partial to a nice blended juice made with different fruits, you'll essentially be consuming high quantities of fructose (fruit sugar) without the neutralizing element of fibre.

While it's true that vegetable juices are also low in fibre, the sugar content is considerably lower and the health benefit is likely to be far greater than in a basic fruit juice. Beetroot juice, for example, has recently been associated with enhanced energy and stamina in athletes. Green juices can be a powerhouse of nutrients, but it's important to watch out for blends that look green, but actually contain several different fruits, such as pineapple, kiwi fruit and apple, with just a small handful of spinach representing the vegetable quota. Even just one apple,

THE RIGHT BITE

A cold-pressed green vegetable juice with a limited amount of fruit to sweeten it is the optimal way to derive the most health benefits from your daily juice, as well as being a quick and easy way of boosting your vegetable intake.

which is a relatively low-sugar fruit, can double the sugar content of a green vegetable juice, and sugary tropical fruits can do an awful lot more damage.

Of course, a vegetable juice of kale, spinach, cucumber, broccoli, herbs, celery or cabbage is going to be packed with vitamin C, B vitamins, iron, magnesium, selenium and zinc, so it can give a much needed boost if you're feeling low.

KEEN JUICERS may want to opt for cold-pressed juice rather than juice from the more common centrifugal juicers, as it's believed that they extract far more of the vitamin and mineral content of the fruit or vegetable.

Coffee Bar

the worst cake scenario

The coffee bar has become an intrinsic part of our daily life in recent years and with it has come a huge increase in our daily caffeine levels, as well as far too many opportunities to top ourselves up with all sorts of little extra treats throughout the week. Coffee bars can be a major trap for the unwary, as cakes, muffins and even healthy-looking oat cookies contain high levels of sugar that will affect your waistline, and if you think having skimmed milk with your latte will help offset that, then think again. Sugar is the key issue here and it's the single biggest culprit when it comes to weight gain (see pages 10–12). Opting for a skinny latte while you tuck into a muffin is really not going to help reduce the inches, if that's your goal.

> Sugar is the single biggest culprit when it comes to weight gain

The other major pitfall of haunting the coffee bar is how much caffeine you're consuming. The maximum recommended amount is 400mg per day and coffee bars vary greatly in the amount of caffeine they offer – anything from 150mg to 400mg per serving, depending on your chosen outlet. Caffeine is a powerful substance and has a major impact on the nervous system, which can lead to sleep problems and that tired-but-wired feeling that you probably know so well. If you're more of a tea drinker, there is no reason to rest on your laurels, as black tea contains roughly 40mg per average cup and for the green tea-lovers among you, be aware that 4 average cups of green tea add up to 100mg of caffeine, roughly the equivalent of a cup of filter coffee.

Many of us rely on caffeine to provide a reliable energy boost to help us cope with our busy daily lives. The irony is that regular caffeine consumption can play a key role in disrupting the energy production process. High levels of caffeine are the enemy of good health: its impact on sleep is well documented, but be aware that excessive caffeine intake can also contribute to high blood pressure and play a part in coronary heart disease.

MUFFINS

The queen of the coffee bar is the muffin – it doesn't matter if you choose a fruit option rather than a chocolate one: either way, you're treading a dangerous path as these are simply stuffed full of sugar. If you've ever made muffins, you'll know that the basic ingredients are sugar, flour, butter (or oil), eggs and milk in some form, and this is never going to be a combination that's kind to your waistline.

However, that's only half the story: mass-produced muffins contain a lot more ingredients, such as thickening agents, stabilizers and vegetable oils, so your favourite muffin could be far more processed than you suspect. In general, the longer the ingredients list, the more processed a product is likely to be.

> **SUGAR CAN BE HIDDEN** on a label in many forms: watch out for any word that ends in '–ose' (e.g. glucose or fructose), honey, syrup, molasses, high fructose corn syrup or hydrolysed starch, as these are all just sugar with another name.

NUTRITION NUMBERS
per unit

↳ FULL-FAT BLUEBERRY MUFFIN
Calories: 448 » Carbohydrate: 43g
Sugars: 28g » Fat: 23g » Fibre: 2g
Protein: 6g

↳ LOW-FAT BLUEBERRY MUFFIN
Calories: 306 » Carbohydrate: 65g
Sugars: 35g » Fat: 2g » Fibre: 2g
Protein: 6g

↳ CHOCOLATE CHIP MUFFIN
Calories: 450 » Carbohydrate: 67g
Sugars: 44g » Fat: 17g » Fibre: 2g
Protein: 6g

↳ BRAN MUFFIN
Calories: 463 » Carbohydrate: 47g
Sugars: 26g » Fat: 24g » Fibre: 5g
Protein: 8g

If you're trying to keep sugar to a minimum, you'd be right in thinking that a chocolate muffin will be higher in added sugar than a blueberry muffin, for example, but there's little difference otherwise, as fruit is still a source of sugar and fruit muffins usually contain generous levels of sugar. It's also worth bearing in mind that cooking the fruit will result in about 25% loss of the vitamin and mineral content, so don't deceive yourself into thinking it's a much healthier option.

It's important to be especially careful if you occasionally allow yourself a low-fat muffin on the basis that it's a moderate treat and a smarter choice than a full-fat muffin. Low-fat foods are actually rather a minefield: as the fat has been stripped out, so has a lot of the flavour, and with that comes extra sugar instead, to compensate. The irony of choosing the low-fat muffin is that in many popular coffee outlets the low-fat version actually contains 2–3 teaspoons of sugar more than the full-fat version, so if you are going to enjoy the occasional treat then you might as well choose the one that tastes better.

THE RIGHT BITE

If you're desperate to have a muffin, then opt for a higher-fibre version. Some outlets stock a breakfast-style muffin that contains oats or bran and nuts and seeds. These tend to be lower in sugar and higher in fibre, keeping you going for longer and minimizing the damage to your waistline.

Full-fat or low-fat, most muffins are a high-sugar snack either way and if you're eating them on a regular basis, you can fully expect to be paying the price in increased inches around the waist.

THE AVERAGE LOW-FAT MUFFIN from a coffee shop contains up to 9 teaspoons of sugar. If you want to do the maths, 4g of sugar is roughly 1 teaspoon. The nutritional information is usually available if you ask, so you can find out in advance whether the low-fat version at your local coffee shop is as 'skinny' as it claims to be.

COOKIES

The basic ingredients of a cookie are not friendly to your waistline, and this isn't helped by the size. A large chocolate chip cookie averages at around 400 calories, which is a costly treat, as it's almost a quarter of the daily recommended calorie intake for women. The high sugar content of a cookie will lead to a blood sugar spike, generating the release of insulin and resulting in a blood sugar crash an hour or two later. This is the danger time, as the cravings will be almost impossible to resist and, before you know it, you'll be reaching for another sugary snack.

Shortbread is a better option, as a standard serving of two small shortbread

A RECENT STUDY SUGGESTED that the processing of oat bran into cookies may reduce the beneficial properties that can help to regulate cholesterol. If you're concerned about your cholesterol levels, you may need to look for less processed ways to incorporate oats into your diet.

NUTRITION NUMBERS
per unit

↳ CHOCOLATE CHIP COOKIE
Calories: 400 » Carbohydrate: 48g
Sugars: 20g » Fat: 18g » Fibre: 1g

↳ SHORTBREAD (per standard pack of 2 small biscuits)
Calories: 200 » Carbohydrate: 31g
Sugars: 12g » Fat: 11g » Fibre: 0.3g

↳ BISCOTTI
Calories: 155 » Carbohydrate: 22g
Sugars: 10g » Fat: 6g » Fibre: 3g

↳ OAT COOKIE
Calories: 300 » Carbohydrate: 45g
Sugars: 24g » Fat: 12g » Fibre: 3g

cookies contains roughly half the amount of sugar of a chocolate chip cookie. Caramel or chocolate chunk shortbread is quite a different matter: if you treat yourself to one of these, then you'll be doubling the calories and consuming the equivalent of 5–6 teaspoons of sugar.

Biscotti are twice-baked Italian biscuits and if you stick with the traditional almond version, rather than the fruity variations, this is a good way to keep your sugar intake under control. Almond biscotti contain about 10g of sugar, which is relatively moderate compared to some of the other cookies on offer. The flour is also mixed with a generous serving of chopped toasted almonds, which adds significantly to the nutrient content by increasing the amount of fibre, vitamins and minerals.

There's usually some form of oat cookie available, which is another way you might be able to limit the damage. These commonly contain some form of dried fruit, which adds to the sugar content, but are likely to be lower in calories and refined sugar than the shortbread or chocolate offerings. Oat cookies have the added benefit

THE RIGHT BITE

Biscotti is the clear winner here, as it's lower in sugar and fat than the other options and even has some residual health benefits to offer with the almond content. If that's not your preferred option, then a carefully chosen oat cookie is likely to be the next best thing – the trick here is to select one that only contains one type of fruit, as this will help to significantly reduce the overall sugar content.

of containing soluble fibre, which will keep you going for longer, as well as promoting optimal digestion and helping to regulate cholesterol levels.

TREATING YOURSELF TO THREE CHOCOLATE CHIP COOKIES over the course of a week adds up to 60g of sugar, which is the equivalent of 15 teaspoons. If you're tucking into cookies on a regular basis, then cutting back on this area alone could make a significant difference to your waistline.

CAKE

A slice of cake is always going to be an indulgence and as any decent cake is going to contain plenty of sugar and butter, it really needs to be an occasional treat or the damage to your waistline will be significant and lasting.

All of the popular options that you find in a coffee shop contain large amounts of sugar, averaging at 32g or 8 teaspoons of sugar per portion, so if you decide to treat yourself to some cake, you need to go into it with your eyes open. When it comes to sugar, fat and calories, there isn't much to choose between coffee shop cakes: brownies, cheesecake and cupcakes are all likely to cause similar

IF YOU THINK THAT A SLICE OF CAKE A WEEK is a moderate approach and a sensible treat, be aware that this adds up to a minimum of 32 teaspoons of sugar over a month. This one small thing could be directly responsible for maintaining a frustratingly stubborn spare tyre.

NUTRITION NUMBERS
per unit

↳ CHOCOLATE BROWNIE
Calories: 350 » Carbohydrate: 34g
Sugars: 28g » Fat: 20g

↳ CARROT CAKE SLICE
Calories: 360 » Carbohydrate: 45g
Sugars: 30g » Fat: 24g

↳ CHEESECAKE SLICE
Calories: 400 » Carbohydrate: 41g
Sugars: 28g » Fat: 27g

↳ CUPCAKE
Calories: 380 » Carbohydrate: 42g
Sugars: 37g » Fat: 20g

↳ LOAF CAKE SLICE
Calories: 380 » Carbohydrate: 45g
Sugars: 38g » Fat: 16g

amounts of damage, although it may come as a surprise to find out that the simple Madeira-style loaf cakes are really no better than the rest. They may appear to be a lighter option, but they often contain more sugar than the other cakes and roughly the same amount of calories, even if they are slightly lower in fat.

As well as adding inches to your waistline, excessive consumption of sugar can exacerbate inflammatory disorders, such as arthritis, joint pain and skin conditions. It may also increase the risk of cardiovascular disease.

The only cake that stands out in nutritional terms is the carrot cake. The average carrot cake contains abut 140g of carrots, which breaks down to about 10g per slice. Carrots are rich in the antioxidant beta carotene, which converts to vitamin A in the body and which is associated with improved night vision and may protect against degenerative eye conditions such as cataracts. Carrots are a good source of vitamins C and E, which are also antioxidants and these help to act against free radicals in the body, which contribute to chronic conditions such as heart disease and certain cancers.

THE RIGHT BITE

When it comes to cake, size matters! The sugar content is high whichever cake you choose, so the smart move is to opt for the smallest slice on offer if cake is a must but you still want to watch your waistline. Sharing it between two, or better still, three people could also help to mitigate the damage.

Encouraging though it sounds, this isn't a reason to get carried away with eating carrot cake, as the amounts of these nutrients are really very small. In any case, the antioxidant effect is likely to be reduced by heating and carrot cake still contains a hefty dose of sugar.

MASS-PRODUCED CAKE often contains trans fats in the form of hydrogenated vegetable oils, as these allow for a longer shelf life. Look out for coffee bars that offer a cake that's hand-baked on the premises, as this is far more likely to be trans fat-free.

PASTRIES

Coffee shops usually offer plenty in the way of sweet pastries. The typical Danish pastry is made with a layered style similar to puff pastry. Anyone familiar with making this type of pastry will know that you need to use vast quantities of butter to achieve the desired effect. Sugar, flour, milk and yeast are the other principal ingredients, so it's unsurprising that the end result contains a hefty calorie count.

Unlike muffins or cookies where it's possible to increase the fibre level and reduce the refined carbohydrates by using wholemeal flour or oats in the mix, recipes for pastries of this sort can't really

SOME COMMERCIALLY PRODUCED PASTRIES use artificial trans fats rather than the traditional butter, as this can extend the shelf life of the product. Trans fats are directly associated with an increased risk of cardiovascular disease and some countries have banned or restricted the use of them in food products.

NUTRITION NUMBERS
per unit

↳ DANISH PASTRY
Calories: 342 » Carbohydrate: 51g
Sugars: 29g » Fat: 14g

↳ CHOCOLATE TWIST
Calories: 334 » Carbohydrate: 45g
Sugars: 20g » Fat: 14g

↳ CINNAMON ROLL
(with dried fruit)
Calories: 381 » Carbohydrate: 65g
Sugars: 27g » Fat: 15g

↳ CREAM SLICE
Calories: 311» Carbohydrate: 31g
Sugars: 20g » Fat: 20g

be successfully adjusted in the same way, if you want to achieve the desired pastry effect. Although there are a number of different styles of pastries on offer in the popular coffee outlets, any buttery pastry product will contain similar proportions of ingredients, so that the nutritional breakdown will be fairly similar, even for a product such as a chocolate twist that seems proportionally smaller.

Whether the topping is icing/confectioner's sugar, honey glaze, fruit puree or dried fruit, these are all forms of sugar which can contribute to the hefty calorie count if one or more feature on your pastry of choice.

There is no getting past the fact that choosing a pastry with your coffee is going to be a high-sugar, high-fat combination that brings a number of potential problems. It's definitely one to avoid if you suffer from any inflammatory conditions, such as arthritis, dermatitis, sinusitis or inflammatory bowel conditions, as both sugar and trans fats are pro-inflammatory and can exacerbate symptoms. Studies have also shown that regularly bingeing on this type of sugar-fat combination

THE RIGHT BITE

Despite the large amounts of butter in pastries, they are comparatively lower in fat than a standard muffin but with the sugar content averaging at 24g across the samples cited opposite, this still adds up to over 6 teaspoons of sugar. Limit your intake to a very occasional treat and share with friends to keep the potential damage to a minimum.

is likely to stimulate an addictive pattern of eating (including withdrawal symptoms) that leads to long-term weight gain.

IT'S IMPORTANT NOT TO MAKE THE MISTAKE of assuming that a pastry that contains dried fruit, such as raisins or sultanas, will automatically be a healthier option. The dehydration process compresses the fruit and concentrates the amount of sugar. Sultanas contain 69g of sugar per 100g, which is more than 17 teaspoons of sugar.

PRETZELS

A pretzel is essentially baked dough, which makes it a starchy option for a snack and it is never going to be a winner when it comes to managing your waistline. However, the good news is that it's likely to be far lower in sugar than many of the other products on offer. In itself, a plain pretzel isn't a terribly interesting offering which is why, in most cases, salt or some other flavouring, such as sugar and/or cinnamon, is added.

The thing to watch out for here is the salt content. Our salt intake is generally far higher than it needs to be, and as it is added to many everyday foods such as bread, cereals and processed food products, it's very easy for salt levels to mount up.

SALT IS NOT ALL BAD and a moderate amount is essential as it plays an important part in muscle function. A deficiency in salt can lead to painful cramps in certain groups of muscles.

NUTRITION NUMBERS
per unit

↳ PLAIN PRETZEL
Calories: 273 » Carbohydrate: 72g
Sugars: 10g » Salt: 0.8g

↳ SALTED PRETZEL
Calories: 330 » Carbohydrate: 60g
Sugars: 6g » Salt: 2g

↳ CINNAMON/SUGARED PRETZEL
Calories: 430 » Carbohydrate: 76g
Sugars: 27g » Salt: 1g

↳ CHOCOLATE PRETZEL
Calories: 482 » Carbohydrate: 81g
Sugars: 28g » Salt: 1g

Excessive levels of salt can disrupt cell function, lead to fluid retention and result in high blood pressure, which is a risk factor for coronary heart disease. Given the amount of salt that's added to our food, a salt deficiency isn't terribly common, but it can explain symptoms such as muscle cramps, headaches and low blood pressure.

Even the 'unsalted' versions of pretzels contain some salt, as it's commonly added to the dough mixture, but the salted pretzel is the one to watch, as it contains roughly 2g of salt, which represents a third of the recommended daily maximum of 6g of salt. If a salted pretzel is a regular treat, then it's worth monitoring your salt consumption for the rest of the day so that you don't overdo it, and it's certainly one to avoid if your blood pressure is a concern.

Opting for a sweet pretzel is immediately going to send the calorie count soaring, and at an average of 430 calories it takes up almost a quarter of the recommended daily calorie intake for women, even though it won't keep you going for very long. Containing roughly 8 teaspoons of sugar per unit,

THE RIGHT BITE

In this case, it depends on your health goal. If you're aiming to lose a spare tyre, then the least sugary option is the salted pretzel. However, if heart health is a concern, the best all-round option is the plain pretzel, as the sugar content is still relatively low (supporting any weight loss goal) and the salt levels are minimal.

it's a direct route to a blood sugar spike. As what goes up must come down, this will be followed by a slump in energy and some serious sugar cravings in a fairly short space of time. This is not a helpful option if you're trying to watch your weight.

DAILY GUIDELINES FOR SALT are to limit adult intake to a maximum of 6g per day. This needs to be reduced for children, depending on their age. Children under the age of one need less than 1g per day.

COFFEE

The levels of caffeine in your coffee can vary dramatically depending on the coffee bar you choose. A medium-size coffee with milk will average at around 150mg of caffeine, but in some places it will be nearer 80mg and in others more than 300mg, which is close to the maximum recommended daily dose of caffeine at 400mg. It's a simple matter to ask the barista or check the coffee bar's website if you're unsure about the caffeine content, because this information should be freely available.

High caffeine levels can impact the body in a number of ways. As a stimulant, caffeine disrupts the nervous system, leading to poor-quality sleep and low energy levels, as well as exacerbating

IF YOU DECIDE TO REDUCE YOUR CAFFEINE CONSUMPTION, then it's important to do so gradually. Going 'cold turkey' can result in unpleasant withdrawal symptoms such as severe headaches, fatigue and aches and pains.

NUTRITION NUMBERS

↳ SINGLE ESPRESSO
Caffeine: 82mg

↳ SMALL CAPPUCCINO/LATTE (240ml)
Caffeine: 102mg
Calories (whole milk): 158
Calories (semi-skimmed milk): 140
Calories (skimmed milk): 74

↳ MEDIUM CAPPUCCINO/LATTE (357ml)
Caffeine: 164mg
Calories (whole milk): 212
Calories (semi-skimmed milk): 188
Calories (skimmed milk): 120

↳ LARGE CAPPUCCINO/LATTE (510ml)
Caffeine: 206mg
Calories (whole milk): 286
Calories (semi-skimmed milk): 250
Calories (skimmed milk): 161

anxiety-related disorders. In sensitive individuals, large amounts of caffeine can lead to an irregular heart beat and may result in high blood pressure. Caffeine can irritate the digestive tract and is best consumed in minimal quantities if you suffer from irritable bowel syndrome or other digestive disorders. It may also increase the rate of bone loss in elderly women. Metabolism of caffeine is a highly individual matter – some people are more affected than others, but if you experience any of these symptoms, you'd be wise to adjust your daily dosage.

On the plus side, the stimulant effect of caffeine can help to increase alertness and mental performance. Some research suggests that drinking coffee regularly may increase longevity and that moderate caffeine consumption on a daily basis may help to reduce the risk of chronic degenerative disease and cognitive decline.

It's not all about the caffeine, however, as there are other pitfalls in the coffee bar. Adding flavoured syrup adds up to 100 calories and a typical caramel-flavoured latte with semi-skimmed milk averages at 300 calories.

THE RIGHT BITE

Small and simple is best – dropping a cup size can make a big difference to the amount of caffeine you're exposed to and sticking to a basic blend of coffee, water and/or milk is likely to be the best way to keep the calories down. The more you add to your coffee in the form of flavoured syrup, whipped cream and chocolate sprinkles, the more empty calories you'll be consuming. A small, skimmed Americano or cappuccino would be a pretty good option.

AS WELL AS CAFFEINE, coffee contains chlorogenic acid and caffeic acid, which have antioxidant properties that may help reduce inflammation and protect against chronic disease. The challenge here is balancing this potential health benefit against the clear disadvantage of consuming excessive levels of caffeine.

TEA

When it comes to tea, the overall caffeine content is lower than coffee, which is a bonus. However, tea-drinkers often consume several cups over the course of a day, which can add up to significant amounts of caffeine. If you're drinking numerous cups of strong tea per day, then this could easily exceed the maximum daily recommendation of 400mg of caffeine so you may want to consider reducing your intake.

Black tea is not the only tea that contains caffeine. In fact, all tea contains caffeine, unless it's a herbal infusion, which will be made very clear on the packaging. Other popular teas, such as

DRINKING A CUP OF TEA WITH A MEAL can impact your iron levels, as tannins found in tea can block the action of non-heme (plant source) iron in the body, which is particularly relevant if you're a vegetarian. Common symptoms of iron deficiency include low energy, headaches and pale skin.

NUTRITION NUMBERS

↳ SMALL CHAI LATTE (240ml)
Caffeine: 70mg
Calories (whole milk): 240
Calories (semi-skimmed milk): 210
Calories (skimmed milk): 185

↳ MEDIUM CHAI LATTE (357ml)
Caffeine: 95mg
Calories (whole milk): 280
Calories (semi-skimmed milk): 260
Calories (skimmed milk): 230

↳ LARGE CHAI LATTE (510ml)
Caffeine: 120mg
Calories (whole milk): 350
Calories (semi-skimmed milk): 320
Calories (skimmed milk): 280

↳ BLACK TEA (per teabag)
Caffeine: 50–75mg (depending on brewing time)

↳ GREEN TEA (per teabag)
Caffeine: 50–75mg (depending on brewing time)

white tea and jasmine tea, still contain caffeine, and even green tea, which is commonly considered to be the healthy option, contains caffeine, so be careful not to overdo it, as this could soon outweigh the health benefits.

Tea contains plant compounds called polyphenols, which are believed to have protective anti-cancer effects. Studies show that green tea is particularly rich in these antioxidants, which offer a range of health benefits, including cardiovascular support and regulating cholesterol levels.

A recent popular addition to the coffee bar is chai latte, a mixture of black tea, spices and milk. This needs to be treated with caution, as it's invariably heavily sweetened with sugar, honey or similar, which is why even the skimmed milk options can be so high in calories.

Herbal teas are actually plant infusions and these don't contain caffeine and don't technically count as a tea. However, they do offer an excellent alternative if you are trying to reduce your caffeine intake and, depending on your choice, have some useful residual health benefits. Peppermint tea can help to soothe unpleasant digestive symptoms

THE RIGHT BITE

Applying a careful balance of black tea and green tea throughout the day could help to ensure you derive the health benefits found in both types of tea, without experiencing the drawbacks of excessive caffeine. Two cups of lightly brewed black tea and two cups of green tea per day add up to roughly 200mg of caffeine, which is much less than you'd find in just one large serving of coffee-shop coffee.

such as bloating or wind; camomile tea calms the nervous system and helps to promote sleep, and liquorice tea provides a useful alternative to dessert and can help to reduce sugar cravings.

THE CAFFEINE CONTENT INCREASES as the tea brews, so the longer you leave the bag in, the stronger it will be: leaving the bag in for 5 minutes more than doubles the caffeine content of tea, compared to 1–2 minutes.

HOT CHOCOLATE

Hot chocolate may seem like a reasonable treat on a cold winter's day but it is actually a major indulgence if you're trying to watch your weight. Whether the base is a processed chocolate powder or genuine melted chocolate, you're setting yourself up for a significant amount of sugar.

Even a small serving of hot chocolate adds up to over 7 teaspoons of sugar and if you decide to treat yourself to a large mug then that's the equivalent of 14 teaspoons of sugar, which is an enormous amount. If you would never dream of drinking a can of standard cola but happily enjoy a large hot chocolate on a regular basis, then be aware that

ADDING WHIPPED CREAM
to your hot chocolate is going to increase the calorie content by at least another 75 calories, so this is definitely one to avoid if you're trying to keep in good shape.

NUTRITION NUMBERS

↳ SMALL (250ml)
Calories (whole milk): 260
Calories (semi-skimmed milk): 201
Calories (skimmed milk): 171
Sugars: 31g » Caffeine: 10mg

↳ MEDIUM (470ml)
Calories (whole milk): 325
Calories (semi-skimmed milk): 290
Calories (skimmed milk): 237
Sugars: 41g » Caffeine: 15mg

↳ LARGE (600ml)
Calories (whole milk): 447
Calories (semi-skimmed milk): 384
Calories (skimmed milk): 335
Sugars: 57g » Caffeine: 20mg

↳ WHIPPED CREAM
(per tablespoon)
Calories: 38 » Carbohydrate: 0.3g
Sugars: 0.3g » Fat: 4g

this adds up to the sugar equivalent of a can and a half of standard cola.

Sugar can also creep into your drink in the form of the various flavoured syrups that are on offer, not to mention the chocolate sprinkles to top it all off. Each shot of flavoured syrup adds the equivalent of 1 teaspoon of sugar to the drink and if you indulge in a generous whipped cream topping, you'll be consuming around another 75 calories, on top of the drink itself. All in all, there are just too many options to add sugar and empty calories to a hot chocolate, which means that it's not something that can sensibly form part of any weight-loss regime.

It's far easier to manage the sugar content of home-made hot chocolate as it is possible to choose a cocoa powder that contains very little or no sugar, although it can taste very bitter as a result. However, when you're out and about there's very little option other than the strongly sweetened versions available. It's also worth bearing in mind that milk is not the problem here, and even if you ask for your hot chocolate drink to be made with water instead of milk, the

sugar content of the chocolate powder remains unchanged.

You may not realize that hot chocolate is a caffeinated drink, even if the caffeine content is relatively low. Unsurprisingly, it depends on the serving size and a large hot chocolate can add up to three-quarters of the caffeine typically found in black tea.

NOT EVERYONE NEEDS TO LOSE WEIGHT and elderly people or those who struggle to take in enough calories could find that a generous mug of hot chocolate is an excellent and easy way to build themselves up.

SMOOTHIES

Smoothies are essentially fruit, usually blended with ice and some form of milk, yogurt or frozen yogurt. As the whole fruit is generally used, helping the drink retain some fibre, smoothies are commonly considered to be preferable to a fruit juice. The fibre content is often minimal, however, and the blades of a blender may damage some of the cellulose in the fruit, reducing the fibre levels.

The real challenge with a smoothie is the amount of sugar it contains, as fruit is full of fructose (fruit sugar), which

FLAXSEED IS A VERY RICH SOURCE OF OMEGA 3 fatty acids and a good alternative if oily fish is not for you. The most robust research into the health benefits for omega 3 is linked to heart health and the regulation of cholesterol levels; however, some studies suggest that it may also help to relieve inflammatory conditions such as arthritis and help to reduce the risk of some cancers.

NUTRITION NUMBERS
per 250ml serving

↳ MANGO & PASSION FRUIT
Calories: 140 » Sugars: 28g
Fibre: 2g

↳ BLUEBERRY & BANANA
Calories: 148 » Sugars: 31g
Fibre: 3g

↳ MIXED FRUITS WITH SEEDS
Calories: 180 » Sugars 30g
Fibre: 4g

↳ PLAIN YOGURT (per 50g)
Calories: 40 » Sugars: 3.5g
Saturated fat: 1g

↳ PLAIN FROZEN YOGURT (per 50g)
Calories: 75 » Sugars: 13g
Saturated fat: 1.5g

can lead to just as much weight gain as classic refined sugar. Every time you enjoy a standard 250ml smoothie, you'll be having the equivalent of at least 7 teaspoons of sugar, roughly the same amount as the average chocolate bar.

Of course, unlike a chocolate bar, assuming your smoothie contains a variety of freshly blended fruit, the micronutrient content of the drink is likely to be high. Fruits such as blueberries, apples and raspberries contain high levels of protective antioxidants, which support the immune system and are believed to help reduce the risk of chronic disease.

However, the high level of sugar means that a blood sugar spike will soon be on the way, leading to sugar cravings. One way to limit the damage would be to choose a smoothie with added protein and fibre, as this can help slow down the release of sugars in the body. Lots of smoothie bars now offer 'super smoothies' that contain flaxseed, chia seeds or other seeds. These are a great source of protein and fibre, as well as containing plenty of omega 3, which plays a key role in heart health.

THE RIGHT BITE

Choosing a smoothie that's a blend of fruit, probiotic yogurt and a generous helping of seeds can transform what is basically a glass full of sugar into a healthy snack that will keep you going for longer and keep the sugar cravings to a minimum.

A final note of caution: check what form of milk is added to your smoothie to create the lovely thick texture. Some contain probiotic yogurt, which helps to promote optimal digestion, but be careful if it contains frozen yogurt, as this often has extra sugar in some form, which will add to the overall calorie count.

CHECK THE SUGAR LEVELS in your favourite smoothie, as it's very important to know exactly how much you're consuming. The average amount of sugar found in a 250ml smoothie is the equivalent amount you would find in a standard chocolate bar, which should give pause for thought.

Working Lunch

mall-nutrition

In a busy working life, lunch can be quite a challenge with only about 10 minutes to rush out, grab something quick and easy and then head back to the desk to eat it. If you're feeling that you deserve something substantial after a tough morning, opting for a carb-heavy lunch can be a serious temptation. Picking the wrong lunch sets you up nicely for the dreaded mid-afternoon slump that leaves you sleepy, unable to concentrate and desperate for a quick energy fix from the cakes and cookies that abound in most office environments.

The single biggest mistake that people make at lunchtime is having too little protein, whether they're virtuously tucking into a leafy green salad concoction or working their way through a hefty baguette sandwich. While meat and fish are excellent sources of protein, it also comes in a range of other guises such as egg, lentils, chickpeas, beans, quinoa, dairy products, nuts and seeds – there are lots of protein options to choose from.

Chewing your food properly triggers the release of digestive enzymes in saliva

Protein is hard to digest and helps to slow down the release of carbohydrate in the body, ensuring sustained energy and helping to reduce mid-afternoon sugar cravings. Eating sufficient quantities of protein can also directly help with weight management. All protein foods contain fats as well, and this is a combination that helps to trigger the satiety mechanism in the body, which tells you that you're full.

Taking the time to eat your lunch mindfully rather than with one hand on the keyboard and both eyes on the screen can also make a major difference to your wellbeing in the afternoon. Chewing your food properly triggers the release of digestive enzymes in saliva that break down carbohydrates and help to generate the satiety response, and it also ensures that large lumps of unchewed food don't pass into the stomach causing bloating and indigestion.

SANDWICHES

When you're pushed for time, a sandwich is the obvious quick and easy option, and if you choose carefully you can achieve a blend of protein and fibre that is likely to keep you going. Unfortunately, it's not always easy to identify the best choice and it's easy to fall victim to the highly refined bread, sugary and fatty sauces or mayonnaise and processed meats that seem to make up the majority of the commercial sandwiches available.

Many sandwiches tend to be pretty stingy on the protein, which means they are not terribly satisfying. This may explain why a sandwich and a packet of potato chips seems to be the standard

IF YOU'VE ALREADY HAD a wheat-based breakfast such as cereal or toast, then a sandwich may not be the best option for you. High levels of wheat with every meal can lead to a sluggish digestion and symptoms of bloating and digestive discomfort, especially in times of stress when your gut is sensitive.

NUTRITION NUMBERS
per sandwich,
with malted white bread

↳ PRAWN/SHRIMP MAYONNAISE
Calories: 305 » Protein: 15g
Carbohydrate: 36g » Sugars: 3g
Fibre: 3g » Total fat: 10g
Saturated fat: 2g

↳ BLT
Calories: 449 » Protein: 21g
Carbohydrate: 45g » Sugars: 6g
Fibre: 4g » Total fat: 20g
Saturated fat: 4g

↳ TUNA MAYONNAISE
Calories: 401 » Protein: 20g
Carbohydrate: 42g » Sugars: 4g
Fibre: 4g » Total fat: 15g
Saturated fat: 1.5g

↳ CHICKEN SALAD
Calories: 414 » Protein: 25g
Carbohydrate: 43g » Sugars: 4g
Fibre: 5g » Total fat: 15g
Saturated fat: 2g

lunch combo for so many people. Made up of over 50% starch, potato chips are a high-carb option so increase the likelihood of a mid-afternoon energy dip. That's before you take into account the perils of deep-fried foods, which increase the risk of chronic disease.

Being picky about the bread that you choose is a good place to start because the more you boost the fibre content of the sandwich, the more satisfying it will be. Opting for wholemeal bread doubles the fibre content and keeps you going for longer, supporting optimal digestion and providing you with energy-boosting B vitamins. Beware of reaching for a chunky baguette sandwich, as this will add roughly another 20% of starchy carbs compared to a standard-size sandwich.

Pay attention to the content of your sandwich to avoid common pitfalls. To minimize saturated fat, opt for lean protein such as chicken, turkey, egg, houmous or salmon rather than cheese, beef or bacon. Meat, fish and eggs are also rich in iron and vitamin B12, which are both essential for optimal energy levels. However, beware of sandwiches with too much mayonnaise, especially the

THE RIGHT BITE

A wholemeal sandwich with lean protein and added salad, rather than just mayonnaise, will provide a much more satisfying option that will limit the potential damage to your waistline and keep you going throughout the afternoon. Aim for a generous portion of lean protein, such as chicken or tuna, with at least two salad vegetables and wholemeal bread to boost fibre levels.

'light' versions. In general these contain double the amount of sugar and salt than standard versions to boost the flavour that has been lost with the removal of the fat.

WATCH OUT FOR TOASTED SANDWICHES AND MELTS – they tend to contain roughly four times the amount of saturated fat as a standard sandwich and fibre levels are minimal, as they rarely come with a wholemeal option and won't contain added fibre in the form of salad.

SALAD

A salad is an obvious healthy choice for lunch and an excellent opportunity to boost vegetable intake to support optimal digestive function and take in plenty of protective antioxidants; however, there are a number of pitfalls for the unwary. The wrong salad can be an unsatisfying lunch that's likely to lead to the mid-afternoon munchies, undoing all your good work. A careless choice of dressing can add up to 300 calories to the meal, making it far from a light option.

USING QUINOA AS A SALAD BASE instead of rice, pasta, noodles or couscous is a great way to boost the protein and fibre levels of your salad. An all-round superfood, quinoa is one of the few plant proteins that contains all the essential amino acids, as well as heart-healthy polyunsaturates. It's also a source of protective antioxidants, and research has shown that quinoa contains plant compounds with anti-inflammatory properties.

NUTRITION NUMBERS
per 300g serving

↳ CHICKEN & PASTA SALAD
Calories: 440 » Protein: 22g
Carbohydrate: 43g » Sugars: 5g
Fat: 16g » Fibre: 4g » Salt: 1g

↳ TUNA NIÇOISE WITH POTATO
Calories: 227 » Protein: 19g
Carbohydrate: 13g » Sugars: 6g
Fat: 10g » Fibre: 4g » Salt: 1g

↳ QUINOA SALAD WITH VEGETABLES & MIXED SEEDS
Calories: 411 » Protein: 22g
Carbohydrate: 42g » Sugars: 5g
Fat: 13g » Fibre: 11g » Salt: 1g

↳ FRENCH DRESSING (per 45g serving)
Calories: 150 » Sugars: 3g
Fat: 14g » Salt: 0.6g

↳ MAYONNAISE (per 45g serving)
Calories: 308 » Sugars: 1g
Fat: 33g » Salt: 0.3g

People who are watching their weight will often opt for green leaves and a few vegetables, assuming that this is the best route to a flat stomach. Unfortunately, the lack of protein means that it's not a terribly sustaining option and is likely to lead to poor food choices further down the line in the form of potato chips, chocolate or biscuits, as the post-lunch slump kicks in.

The other common error with choosing a salad is to pick a pasta or noodle-based option, on the assumption that this will keep you going. It will add a hefty serving of refined carbohydrate, as it's rare to have wholegrain pasta or noodles on offer. The body will burn quickly through the refined carbohydrate, so you're likely to experience a blood sugar crash mid-afternoon and be desperate for a quick sugary fix.

A vegetable-rich salad is a healthy option, and a generous portion of green leaves, such as spinach, rocket/arugula or watercress, will provide optimal levels of magnesium, helping to calm the nervous system and regulating the body's response to stress. To make it into a satisfying meal, ensure that a quarter of the salad is made up of protein.

THE RIGHT BITE

A salad packed with a range of fibrous vegetables and a generous source of protein (ideally about a quarter of the overall salad), such as meat, fish, egg, houmous, quinoa or lentils, is the best way to ensure you're getting the most out of your lunch. Avoiding commercial salad dressings, which can be high in empty calories, sugars and preservatives, is also a smart move – a simple mixture of olive oil and balsamic vinegar can add flavour without doing so much damage.

BEWARE LOW-FAT MAYONNAISE – it may seem like the healthier option but it contains roughly double the amount of sugar and salt per serving of regular mayonnaise. Sugary options, such as sweet chilli dressing, are also best avoided, as a 45ml serving can add over 250 calories to your salad.

SOUP

A carefully chosen soup can offer a highly nutritious lunch and it can be an easy and painless way to increase your vegetable intake, if this is an area you find challenging. It's important to choose a soup that is rich in protein, as the popular options of tomato or mixed vegetable soup may seem a virtuous choice in the short term but in the long term, they're likely to have you reaching for a snack mid-afternoon, as it's simply not enough to keep you going.

Soups made with plant protein such as lentils, chickpeas or beans are an excellent option, as these pulses are also full of fibre, offering the ideal balance of nutrients to maintain blood sugar

WATCH OUT FOR THE SALT CONTENT of processed soups, especially canned or add-water versions, as these can be surprisingly high in salt compared to the soup found in fresh cartons. A high salt intake contributes to fluid retention and high blood pressure.

NUTRITION NUMBERS
per 350g serving of fresh soup

↳ TOMATO
Calories: 171 » Protein: 3g
Fat: 7g » Sugars: 14g
Fibre: 3g » Salt: 1.5g

↳ CARROT & CORIANDER
Calories: 185 » Protein: 3g
Fat: 9g » Sugars: 11g
Fibre: 5g » Salt: 1.2g

↳ LENTIL & TOMATO
Calories: 241 » Protein: 13g
Fat: 4g » Sugars: 10g
Fibre: 4g » Salt: 1.2g

↳CHICKEN & VEGETABLE
Calories: 245 » Protein: 11g
Fat: 11g » Sugars: 8g
Fibre: 4g » Salt: 1.7g

↳ SPICY CHICKPEA & VEGETABLE
Calories: 285 » Protein: 13g
Fat: 7g » Sugars: 11g
Fibre: 7g » Salt: 1g

levels and ensure sustained energy. They also have the added bonus of heart-healthy polyunsaturated fats as well as containing plant compounds that promote hormone balance.

The temptation with soup can be to have a hefty helping of bread to make the dish more satisfying and this is where lots of damage can be done. If your taste runs to a crusty baguette, this will add significant amounts of refined starch to the meal, sending blood sugar levels high and setting you up for the dreaded mid-afternoon slump later. If ruling out bread is not an option, then choose a high-fibre bread such as wholemeal, seeded or rye. These will keep you going for far longer than refined white breads.

Studies have shown that eating soup regularly can help to promote weight loss, as the blend of nutrients and water in chicken and vegetable soup, for example, slows down gastric emptying and stays in the stomach for longer, compared to a meal of chicken with vegetables. As you feel fuller for longer, this encourages the reduction of ghrelin, a hormone that plays a part in stimulating the appetite.

THE RIGHT BITE

A protein-rich soup is always going to be the most satisfying option. Some meat-based soups can be surprisingly stingy on the protein, as meat is an expensive ingredient, whereas soups made with cost-effective pulses such as beans, lentils or chickpeas often contain more generous proportions of protein. Aim for a portion that contains a minimum of 9g of protein and if you can find a soup that combines meat with pulses, then you're onto a winner as this is a fool-proof way to boost your protein levels.

ALL SOUPS CAN HELP WITH A WEIGHT-MANAGEMENT PROGRAMME as the water helps it stay in the stomach for longer, but studies have shown that smooth, blended soups win out over chunky soups when it comes to inducing a sense of fullness. Getting busy with the blender could make all the difference to keeping you in shape.

SUSHI & SASHIMI

The classic sushi box has much to recommend it, as it's full of lean protein and omega 3 fatty acids, with some hidden benefits along the way, such as ginger, nori and wasabi. In general, the mineral content of raw fish is higher than cooked fish, which is a bonus, but there is also the potential issue of marine contaminants, such as mercury or other heavy metals, to consider. These can be stored in the flesh of larger fish, such as tuna, which is why only small quantities are advised for pregnant women, the elderly or other vulnerable groups.

Nigri – strips of raw salmon or tuna on a bed of white rice prepared with

> **USING THE WHOLE SOY BEAN** in the form of edamame beans, rather than the processed forms of soy foods that are so common in the West, is far preferable, as the documented health benefits of soy relate to the wholefood form.

NUTRITION NUMBERS
per 4 units

↳ VEGETABLE MAKI ROLL
Calories: 113 » Protein: 4g
Carbohydrate: 17g » Fibre: 2g
Fat: 3g » Salt: 0.8g

↳ TUNA MAKI ROLL
Calories: 115 » Protein: 8g
Carbohydrate: 14g » Fibre: 1g
Fat: 1g » Salt: 1g

↳ SALMON NIGRI
Calories: 126 » Protein: 8g
Carbohydrate: 13g » Fibre: 0.5g
Fat: 5g » Salt: 0.6g

↳ CRAB CALIFORNIA ROLL
Calories: 127 » Protein: 5g
Carbohydrate: 16g » Fibre: 4g
Fat: 3g » Salt: 0.7g

↳ EDAMAME (per 100G)
Calories: 125 » Protein: 9g
Carbohydrate: 11g » Fibre: 6g
Fat: 4g » Salt: 0.02g

vinegar – are a good option. The sticky white sushi rice is a high-starch option, but the portions are usually fairly small and the overall nutritional profile of the dish offers quite a bit of compensation in the way of lean protein and heart-healthy omega 3 fatty acids. Some outlets prepare brown rice sushi, which is always going to be the optimal option, as it boosts fibre content and, coupled with the lean protein of the fish, is the ideal blood sugar-balancing lunch.

Maki rolls don't pack the same health punch as nigri – canned fish is commonly used here, which dramatically reduces the omega 3 content compared to using fresh fish. The vegetarian options lack protein so they're not a very sustaining lunch and are likely to leave you open to the munchies later in the afternoon.

The extras that accompany sushi have some surprising advantages. For example, the seaweed (nori) that wraps maki rolls is one of the rare food sources of iodine, which plays an essential role in optimal thyroid function. Seaweed is also considered to have anti-inflammatory properties and to reduce PMS symptoms by supporting hormone balance.

THE RIGHT BITE

The ideal combination is a selection of nigri with a serving of edamame beans and salad, which is a common offering in lots of outlets. This way you derive all the benefit of the lean protein and omega 3 in the nigri, while the fibre content of the beans and salad will help to neutralize the effect of the starchy white rice, if a brown rice version isn't available.

Adding a generous serving of ginger when you prepare your nigri is also a good idea. Ginger has a range of health benefits, such as relieving symptoms of nausea and supporting optimal digestion. It also has antimicrobial properties that may support optimal immune function.

SOME STUDIES HAVE SHOWN that spicy green wasabi paste contains sulphur compounds that may help to protect against the growth of cancer cells.

RICE & NOODLE POTS

A spicy noodle or rice pot has the potential to be a very satisfying lunch. It's worth taking the time to make a judicious choice as this can make all the difference between sustained energy and a spring in your step all afternoon, rather than the yawning lethargy of the post-lunch slump.

First pay attention to the size of the rice or noodle portion as it can often be excessive and certainly shouldn't exceed one-third (preferably one-quarter) of the pot; if it's also white rice or noodles, you're heading for trouble. This is a large

PAY PARTICULAR ATTENTION to the accompanying sauces – if the dish is cooked in a simple miso-style broth, this will do considerably less damage than some of the popular sauces that get ladled over the rice or noodles. A modest portion of 50ml (which isn't a lot) of sweet & sour sauce contains more than 3 teaspoons of sugar.

NUTRITION NUMBERS
per 100g (cooked)

↳ WHITE RICE
Calories: 131 » Carbohydrate: 31g
Fibre: 0.5g

↳ BROWN RICE
Calories: 132 » Carbohydrate: 29g
Fibre: 3g

↳ WHITE NOODLES
Calories: 166 » Carbohydrate: 36g
Fibre: 1g

↳ WHOLEGRAIN NOODLES
Calories: 174 » Carbohydrate: 35g
Fibre: 3g

SAUCES per 50ml serving

↳ SWEET & SOUR SAUCE
Calories: 58 » Sugars: 13g

↳ TERIYAKI SAUCE
Calories: 66 » Sugars: 11g

↳ SWEET CHILLI SAUCE
Calories: 53 » Sugars: 10g

serving of refined carbohydrate that won't do your waistline or your energy levels any favours. Check if your favourite outlet has whole-wheat noodles and brown rice on offer, as this will keep you going for far longer than the refined white versions.

However, if you struggle with IBS-type symptoms, especially at times of stress, opt for rice rather than noodles, as high levels of dietary wheat can act as an irritant to a sensitive digestive tract. Bear in mind that egg noodles are also made from wheat, so you would need to opt for wheat-free buckwheat or rice noodles, if reducing wheat is a consideration and you don't enjoy rice.

Brown rice offers a range of other residual health benefits: not only is it an excellent source of both soluble and insoluble fibre that helps to promote optimal digestion, but the presence of soluble fibre and rice bran oil can help to regulate cholesterol levels. The low glycaemic index (GI) of brown rice may also explain why regular consumption is associated with a reduced risk of obesity and type 2 diabetes.

Ideally, your rice or noodle pot should feature a generous portion of protein,

THE RIGHT BITE

Opting for brown rice rather than noodles, along with a generous serving of vegetables and lean protein, such as chicken, will tick all the boxes for optimal digestion, sustained energy and weight management. Keeping sugary sauces to a minimum will also help to retain the low GI element of the meal.

such as lean meat, fish, lentils or tofu, along with a range of fibrous vegetables. By balancing your meal carefully in this way, blood sugar levels will be maintained, ensuring sustained energy throughout the afternoon as well as helping to boost your five-a-day.

BROWN RICE IS AN EXCELLENT SOURCE OF MAGNESIUM, a mineral that plays a key part in a number of areas, such as regulating blood pressure, contributing to bone health and supporting optimal function of the nervous system.

Takeout and Fast Food

fries, pies and lies

Whether it's a regular guilty pleasure or an emergency measure when you're out and about, fast food needs to be treated with caution if you want to keep things healthy. Some fast food outlets have worked hard in recent years at including healthy offerings such as salads, but the reality is that you don't usually go to one of these places for a salad. So what are the pitfalls when it comes to your favourite takeout food and how can you limit the potential damage?

Much depends on what your health concern might be. Fast food tends to be high in sugar and refined carbohydrate (leading to weight gain), trans fats (increasing the risk of heart disease) and salt (impacting on blood pressure).

Whether your taste runs to burgers, fried chicken, pizza, Chinese or Indian food, there is no getting away from the fact that much of it can be highly processed, so it should really only be consumed as an occasional treat. And, for the record, a treat is 'an event or item that is out of the ordinary' and not something you have 2-3 times a week. That's a habit, not a treat!

Carefully selected Indian, Chinese and Tex Mex food contains some surprising health benefits

However, if you do want to let go and enjoy some takeout food, then smart choices can really help. It is possible to join in with friends and family and enjoy a pizza or a burger while limiting the potential damage to your waistline, while carefully selected Indian, Chinese and Tex Mex food contains some surprising health benefits.

It's not just about careful menu choices, though – your choice of outlet plays a major part. The standard of the meat can vary greatly from quality cuts, locally sourced, to a blend of fatty cuts, connective tissue and sinew. Do you actually know what you're eating and where it comes from? If you want to benefit from meat that contains appropriate levels of lean protein, vitamins and minerals, then it might be worth asking the question or finding out more from the outlet's website.

BURGERS

Beef is an excellent source of protein, which is essential for growth and repair of body cells, including skin healing, muscle building, and strengthening hair and nails. This is a very good reason to ensure that you choose your burger with care. Burger meat can vary greatly in quality, with cheaper burgers often containing sinew and connective tissue, which is neither appetizing nor good for you. In recent years there has been a gradual move toward using beef from grass-fed rather than grain-fed cattle and this is believed to increase the levels of omega 3 fatty acids in the meat. Finding out about the provenance of the beef from your preferred outlet can help you find out if you're maximizing your health options.

IF YOU TREAT YOURSELF to a large burger, medium fries and a medium cola, that adds up to almost 1,000 calories, which is half the daily recommended allowance for women and doesn't leave you much for the rest of the day.

NUTRITION NUMBERS

↳ BASIC HAMBURGER
Calories: 260 » Protein: 14g
Carbohydrate: 30g » Sugars: 7g
Saturated fat: 4g » Salt: 1.3g

↳ BASIC CHEESEBURGER
Calories: 305 » Protein: 17g
Carbohydrate: 31g » Sugars: 7g
Saturated fat: 7g » Salt: 1.8g

↳ DELUXE HAMBURGER
WITH CHEESE
Calories: 550 » Protein: 30g
Carbohydrate: 45g » Sugars: 11g
Saturated fat: 13g » Salt: 2.5g

↳ CHICKEN BURGER IN A
WHOLEMEAL BUN
Calories: 400 » Protein: 28g
Carbohydrate: 45g » Sugars: 5g
Saturated fat: 2g » Salt: 2g

↳ FRIES (medium serving)
Calories: 323 » Carbohydrate: 43g
Saturated fat: 2.5g » Total fat: 15g

Some of the chicken or fish burgers are interesting options, as they are leaner and the saturated fat content is about five times lower. A deluxe hamburger with cheese commonly contains over half the daily recommended amount of saturated fat, which is a lot to take in at one sitting, especially if heart health is a concern.

The other main challenge of enjoying a burger is that it's not just about the meat – you're contending with highly refined carbohydrate in the form of the bun. The average burger bun is far sweeter than normal bread and contains roughly 2 teaspoons of added sugar as well as refined white flour – a nice package of sugar that goes straight to your waistline.

Watch out for the sauces, too: 30% of tomato ketchup is just sugar, so if you're piling this on liberally, it won't help matters. Some of the 'special' burger sauces contain high fructose corn syrup, a highly processed form of sugar that goes directly to your liver and which is considered to be the principal factor behind fatty liver disease, which affects 90 million Americans.

If your blood pressure level is a concern, keep an eye on salt intake. The average burger contains up to 3g of salt, which is half the recommended daily allowance in just one quick meal.

THE RIGHT BITE

If you're eating in, then there is often the option to have a 'naked' burger, which means no bun, just the burger and the trimmings, missing out on a lot of empty calories. If you're taking away, then keep it simple, as a basic hamburger contains far less sugar, saturated fat and calories than the deluxe version. If you can find one of the elusive wholemeal buns on offer, that will keep you going for longer and reduce the chances of getting the munchies later.

KEEPING FRIES TO A MINIMUM is a smart move – a medium portion doubles the overall calorie count and large fries add up to 439 calories, more than most of the burgers on offer. Small fries are 230 calories per portion.

PIZZA

Unsurprisingly, pizza can be high in calories, full of starch, fat and salt, and has a number of potential pitfalls, depending on the topping.

Pepperoni and spicy sausage pizzas need to be treated with caution. These highly processed meats are loaded with salt, artificial flavourings and preservatives, such as nitrates, which may trigger migraines in sensitive individuals. High levels of salt contribute to high blood pressure – just 3 slices of pepperoni or spicy sausage pizza exceeds the recommended daily limit for salt.

IF YOU REGULARLY TUCK INTO a whole large deep pan pizza then you'll be consuming an average of 2,000 calories, before you take into account any little extras such as garlic bread, sugary drinks or alcohol. Even a large thin crust pizza is likely to take you over 1,500 calories, so when you're eating pizza, less is definitely best if you want to keep the calories down.

NUTRITION NUMBERS
per slice of a large pizza

↳ DEEP PAN PEPPERONI
Calories: 306 » Carbohydrate: 27g
Sugars: 3g » Saturated fat: 6g
Protein: 13g » Salt: 2g

↳ THIN CRUST PEPPERONI
Calories: 219 » Carbohydrate: 19g
Sugars: 2g » Saturated fat: 5g
Protein: 10g » Salt: 2g

↳ DEEP PAN 'MEATY'
Calories: 340 » Carbohydrate: 27g
Sugars: 3g » Saturated fat: 6g
Protein: 17g » Salt: 3g

↳ THIN CRUST 'MEATY'
Calories: 262 » Carbohydrate: 20g
Sugars: 2g » Saturated fat: 5g
Protein: 12g » Salt: 3g

↳ DEEP PAN VEGETARIAN
Calories: 225 » Carbohydrate: 29g
Sugars: 3g » Saturated fat: 3g
Protein: 10g » Salt: 2g

→ THIN CRUST VEGETARIAN
Calories: 163 » Carbohydrate: 20g
Sugars: 2g » Saturated fat: 2g
Protein: 9g » Salt: 1g

The biggest challenge with pizza is the impact on your waistline, as few people stop at just one slice. Tucking into 3 slices of deep pan pepperoni pizza equals over 900 calories. Much of this is due to a generous serving of cheese and a high level of carbs in the base – 3 slices add up to 81g of carbs, the rough equivalent of 5 slices of bread. A thin crust version can help to keep the carb levels down, but does little to limit the high levels of saturated fat. Three slices of a meaty pizza will add up to 15g (thin crust) or 18g (deep pan) of saturated fat – very close to the guideline daily amount of 20g.

A vegetarian pizza is likely to be lower in saturated fat and salt. Adding peppers, mushrooms, onions or spinach can make a big difference, boosting the fibre content to help neutralize excess sugar in the base, and adding a few antioxidants, B vitamins and magnesium, to support immune function and increase energy levels.

THE RIGHT BITE

The simpler your pizza, the less alarming the nutrition numbers are likely to be. Opting for a thin crust vegetarian pizza can dramatically reduce the calorie, carb and fat count of your meal. If vegetarian is not an option for you, then aim for a simple pizza – choosing a basic ham and mushroom pizza with a thin crust base can roughly halve the calories and limit the exposure to processed meat. Some pizza outlets offer 'pizza-light', a lower-calorie thin crust option served with salad, which is a great way to join in with everyone without doing too much damage.

ORDERING A DOUBLE PORTION
of jalapeño chilli peppers can have an anti-inflammatory effect – the hotter the pepper, the more capsaicin it contains, which acts as a natural painkiller and may provide some relief from joint pain and arthritic conditions.

FRIED CHICKEN

Fried chicken is shockingly high in calories and saturated fat and a large sharing portion can do a lot of damage. Sharing food often means that you eat more than you usually would, and you could easily find yourself putting away over half of the daily recommended amount of calories.

There's a vast difference between chicken nuggets sold in burger bars and a classic fried chicken portion. A box of chicken nuggets weighs about 250g (less than just one fried chicken thigh or breast), which is why the calorie count is significantly lower. The batter on a nugget is also far less thick than a deep-fried wing or drumstick, for example.

TREAT DIP POTS WITH CAUTION – a basic barbecue sauce pot is roughly 50 calories, a sweet chilli dip pot is 75 calories and if you opt for honey mustard or ranch cream dip, you'll be adding up to 130 calories.

NUTRITION NUMBERS

↳ CLASSIC FRIED CHICKEN
1 drumstick
Calories: 137 » Carbohydrate: 4g
Saturated fat: 2g » Protein: 12g
Salt: 1g

1 thigh
Calories: 295 » Carbohydrate: 7g
Saturated fat: 5g » Protein: 19g
Salt: 2g

1 breast
Calories: 310 » Carbohydrate: 12g
Saturated fat: 4g » Protein: 36g
Salt: 3g

1 wing
Calories: 117 » Carbohydrate: 5g
Saturated fat: 1g » Protein: 10g
Salt: 1g

↳ CHICKEN NUGGETS (box of 6)
Calories: 275 » Carbohydrate: 21g
Saturated fat: 2.5g » Protein: 12g
Salt: 2g

However, despite the lower calorie count, chicken nuggets are often made up of a blend of component parts of the chicken, which can include connective tissue and fat, whereas classic fried chicken uses a recognized cut, such as thigh or breast.

Just 4 pieces of fried chicken in a variety box add up to almost 900 calories, and that's before any fries, drinks or desserts, so you need to be mindful of the potential damage to your waistline. The quality of the product can also vary dramatically across the different outlets, as much will depend on the suppliers of the chicken and the cooking methods of the store.

Do you know if the chicken you're eating is intensively farmed or free-range? This can have a significant impact on the quality. It's not uncommon for suppliers to inject chicken with water or protein to increase the size and weight of the product. The quality of the cooking oil is another major factor – the more it is reused the more likely it is to become rancid and to develop free radicals, which can cause cell damage and increase the risk of developing certain cancers.

THE RIGHT BITE

Ideally, the chicken shouldn't be fried at all – some outlets offer a grilled version, which can knock off around 100 calories from breast or thighs and around 50 calories from drumsticks and wings. It also halves the saturated fat content, which is quite significant. If this isn't for you, then you could try opting for the lower-calorie/fat versions by eating more drumsticks and wings and fewer breast and thighs. Stripping off some of the batter and just eating the chicken will also help to limit the damage.

EATING LARGE QUANTITIES OF DEEP-FRIED FOOD, which is usually highly processed, is associated with an increased risk of cardiovascular diseases, such as atherosclerosis (fatty deposits in the arteries). By opting for 4 pieces of breast or thigh, rather than a variety of pieces, you could reach the daily recommended maximum for saturated fat of 20g in just one meal.

FISH & CHIPS

Traditionally, white fish, such as cod, haddock or plaice, is used for fish and chips and although these lack the high levels of omega 3 found in oily fish, such as salmon or tuna, they still contain plenty of goodness. White fish is full of lean protein and low in saturated fat, as well as being a useful source of B vitamins and iron, which are both important for energy production. White fish is also rich in selenium, a mineral that's essential for thyroid function, enhances sperm production and motility, and is a powerful antioxidant believed to protect against some cancers.

The problems start when you dip the fish in batter and deep-fry it, as this is when the calorie and fat content increases significantly. The thickness of

THE THICKNESS OF THE CHIPS can also contribute to the fat content, as thicker chips seem to absorb more fat than thin-cut chips, possibly due to the fact that they need to be cooked for longer.

NUTRITION NUMBERS

↳ COD SMALL (110g)
Calories: 247 » Carbohydrate: 13g
Saturated fat: 9g » Protein: 16g

↳ COD MEDIUM (170g)
Calories: 269 » Carbohydrate: 16g
Saturated fat: 11g » Protein: 18g

↳ COD LARGE (280g)
Calories: 291 » Carbohydrate: 20g
Saturated fat: 14g » Protein: 20g

↳ CHIPS SMALL (140g)
Calories: 312 » Carbohydrate: 31g
Saturated fat: 7g

↳ CHIPS MEDIUM (280g)
Calories: 596 » Carbohydrate: 84g
Saturated fat: 13g

↳ CHIPS LARGE (425g)
Calories: 902 » Carbohydrate: 127g
Saturated fat: 19g

↳ MUSHY PEAS (85g serving)
Calories: 81 » Carbohydrate: 14g
Protein: 5.8g

the batter and the portion sizes will vary dramatically across the different outlets, so it's important to find out the weight of the food you're choosing, as this can have a big impact on the nutritional profile of your meal. While fish and chips is never likely to be the lowest calorie option, it is possible to mitigate the damage to your waistline by thinking carefully about the portion size: a large cod and chips adds up to over 1,000 calories, so just by having a large cod and small chips, you could almost halve the overall calories of the meal.

If you're concerned about the fat content of your chips, then it's worth noting that beef dripping, for example, is far higher in fat than rapeseed or palm oil. The quality of the fat can also have a health impact – oil that has been reused over a long period of time can become rancid, developing free radicals that can cause cell damage.

As with all deep-fried foods, there is the ongoing concern of the increased risk of inflammatory conditions such as cardiovascular disease, high cholesterol and obesity if you're regularly eating large quantities. Recent studies have also shown that regular consumption of deep-fried foods – more than twice per week – may increase the risk of certain cancers.

THE RIGHT BITE

It's all about the size and proportions: more fish and fewer chips will make a significant difference to the fat and carbohydrate content of the meal, because the chip portion is where the main damage is done. It also means you make the most of all the beneficial nutrients in the fish, while limiting the empty calories of the chips. If you can eat the fish and leave the batter, this will help to reduce the saturated fat content further.

NOT ALL THE LITTLE EXTRAS ARE EQUAL: mushy peas are a great addition to your meal, as they're virtually fat-free and are a good source of protein. However, if you're partial to a generous serving of curry sauce on your chips, watch out, as this is just a large helping of roughly 150 empty calories.

DONER KEBAB

The doner kebab, shawarma or gyro are all basically the same thing: slivers of spicy meat served in a pitta with salad. On the face of it, this should be a fairly harmless offering but there's more to this simple snack than meets the eye.

The meat (which is usually lamb, but can be chicken, beef or even goat) is prepared by alternating strips of fat with meat and building it around a rotating skewer or spit and then served by shaving off slices of cooked meat. This explains why a single medium-size kebab contains 150% of the guideline daily amount of saturated fat and why it is so high in calories, adding up to over 1,000 calories per unit. If you're tucking

RECENT RESEARCH INTO THE CONTENT OF DONER KEBABS revealed that there was little difference in weight between serving sizes labelled 'small' or 'large', so ordering a small kebab is unlikely to help to significantly keep the calories down.

NUTRITION NUMBERS
per medium-size kebab

↳ MEAT (200g)
Calories: 754 » Total fat: 63g
Saturated fat: 31g » Protein: 47g
Salt: 4g

↳ PITTA
Calories: 255 » Total fat: 1g
Saturated fat: 0g » Protein: 9g
Salt: 1g

↳ SALAD
Calories: 95 » Total fat: 0g
Saturated fat: 0g » Protein: 1g
Salt: 0g

↳ WHOLE KEBAB
Calories: 1104 » Total fat: 64g
Saturated fat: 31g » Protein: 57g
Salt: 5g

↳ SHISH KEBAB WITH PITTA AND SALAD (per 250g serving)
Calories: 372 » Total fat: 10g
Saturated fat: 4g » Protein: 32g
Salt: 2g

into a kebab after a few beers, then this night out is guaranteed to add inches to your waistline.

The large amount of fat in a kebab is the main reason for the excessive calorie count, and this is calculated before any potentially high-calorie additions such as mayonnaise, chilli and garlic sauce or ketchup, which often contain surprising amounts of sugar.

Salt is another area of concern, as the average kebab contains almost the entire daily guideline limit for salt, which means you need to be very careful about your salt intake for the rest of the day. There's no denying that such a high-calorie mix of saturated fat and salt on a regular basis should lead to warning bells – if you're enjoying a kebab on a regular basis, it's a fast route to a number of health risks, such as obesity, high blood pressure and cardiovascular disease.

The quality of the meat and the size of the serving can vary greatly from one outlet to the next. Food and safety inspections have revealed that the kebab meat in some outlets is made up of meat from a variety of different animals and that this is not always highlighted

THE RIGHT BITE

There's no way around the fact that a doner kebab is not a terribly healthy takeout option. Swapping to a shish kebab could make all the difference, as this uses whole cuts of meat grilled on a skewer before being added to a pitta. This can cut the calorie count by roughly half and contains about a quarter of the saturated fat of a doner kebab.

to customers. This presents potential cultural and religious issues, as well as possible health concerns. Make sure you ask the question of your favourite kebab shop, if you want to be sure that you know exactly what you're eating when you buy a doner kebab.

MANY OF THE MOST POPULAR ADDED EXTRAS can have some hidden pitfalls: a standard serving of ketchup or chilli and garlic sauce contain 1.5 teaspoons of sugar, so watch out if you're ladling it on.

TEX MEX

The challenge with tacos and burritos is that it's a build-your-own meal – the basic starting ingredients add up to 400–500 calories but if you get carried away with your other choices then it's easy to make the whole thing add up to more than 1,000 calories.

Watch out for the refined carbohydrate of the floury tortilla and white rice, which will soon add inches to your waistline. The smart move is to focus on including nutrient-dense toppings that will keep you going for longer and that have some residual health benefits along the way.

Brown rice triples the amount of available fibre, providing more sustained energy than white rice, as well as being a great source of energy-boosting B vitamins and magnesium. If you opt

AVOCADO CONTAINS a wide range of carotenoids, powerful antioxidants with anti-inflammatory properties, which are believed to help promote heart health and reduce the risk of chronic disease.

NUTRITION NUMBERS
served with cheese and salad

↳ BEEF TACO
Calories: 437 » Carbohydrate: 34g
Sugars: 4g » Fibre: 6g » Salt: 0.8g
Saturated fat: 5g » Protein: 32g

↳ CHICKEN TACO
Calories: 401 » Carbohydrate: 32g
Sugars: 3g » Fibre: 7g » Salt: 0.7g
Saturated fat: 4g » Protein: 33g

↳ BEEF BURRITO
Calories: 512 » Carbohydrate: 52g
Sugars: 1g » Fibre: 4g » Salt: 3g
Saturated fat: 7g » Protein: 42g

↳ CHICKEN BURRITO
Calories: 497 » Carbohydrate: 49g
Sugars: 0g » Fibre: 4g » Salt: 3g
Saturated fat: 6g » Protein: 44g

↳ NAKED CHICKEN BURRITO
Calories: 289 » Carbohydrate: 2g
Sugars: 0g » Fibre: 1.5g » Salt: 1.3g
Saturated fat: 8g » Protein: 39g

TOPPINGS

↳ GUACAMOLE (80g)

Calories: 204 » Carbohydrate: 7g
Sugars: 1g » Fibre: 5g » Salt: 0.83g
Saturated fat: 3g » Protein: 2g

↳ BEANS (100g)

Calories: 118 » Carbohydrate: 20g
Sugars: 1g » Fibre: 10g » Salt: 0.75g
Saturated fat: 0g » Protein: 6g

↳ SOUR CREAM (50g)

Calories: 117 » Carbohydrate: 1g
Sugars: 2g » Fibre: 0g » Salt: 0.08g
Saturated fat: 7g » Protein: 2g

↳ WHITE RICE (100g)

Calories: 187 » Carbohydrate: 34g
Sugars: 0g » Fibre: 1g » Salt: 0.9g
Saturated fat: 0g » Protein: 3g

for beans then this is an ideal blend of protein and fibre, which helps to maintain blood sugar levels and reduce sugar cravings. Beans are rich in soluble fibre, which helps to regulate cholesterol levels and they also contain

THE RIGHT BITE

The optimal choice is clear – a naked burrito means that you lose the highly refined tortilla, which virtually wipes out the refined carbohydrate content and knocks 200 empty calories off the dish straight away. If the tortilla is a must-have, then choose beans, guacamole and brown rice as your extras; this can still make it a nutritious meal, which should keep you going for hours, and ticks all the boxes for heart health.

plant compounds with hormone-balancing properties.

Guacamole is another excellent option. There is a tendency to avoid avocado as it's high in fat, but 75% of the fat is made up of healthy mono- and polyunsaturated fats that have a number of health benefits associated with reducing the risk of heart disease. If you want to keep saturated fat to a minimum, then limit yourself to cheese or sour cream, rather than having both, and choose chicken over beef.

INDIAN FOOD

Indian food consists of a wide range of dishes usually made from lean, spicy meat or fish and a range of vegetables and pulses. The base of almost every dish involves garlic, ginger and turmeric, which have several health benefits. Other common herbs and spices include cardamom and coriander, which support optimal digestion and have anti-bacterial properties, which is all good news, so far.

Unfortunately, many of the dishes commonly found on Indian takeaway menus have been adapted to Western tastes and include creamy, sugary sauces that are a far cry from what you'd find in India. There is also a strong focus on accompanying starch in the form of large

ANTI-INFLAMMATORY TURMERIC, which is a key component of most Indian dishes, helps to protect against cell damage in the liver, so enjoying a turmeric-rich Indian takeout may not be such a bad idea after an extended session at the pub.

NUTRITION NUMBERS
per 350g serving

↳ CHICKEN KORMA
Calories: 605 » Carbohydrate: 21g
Sugars: 13g » Saturated fat: 14g
Protein: 44g » Salt: 2g

↳ LAMB ROGAN JOSH
Calories: 435 » Carbohydrate: 20g
Sugars: 13g » Saturated fat: 6g
Protein: 33g » Salt: 2g

↳ MEAT CURRY
Calories: 507 » Carbohydrate: 9g
Sugars: 4g » Saturated fat: 10g
Protein: 40g » Salt: 1g

↳ HALF A NAAN BREAD (100g)
Calories: 285 » Carbohydrate: 50g
Sugars: 3g » Saturated fat: 1g
Protein: 8g » Salt: 1.5g

↳ PILAU RICE (100g)
Calories: 142 » Carbohydrate: 25g
Sugars: 1g » Saturated fat: 3g
Protein: 2g » Salt: 1g

amounts of rice and naan bread, which can almost double the calorie count of your chosen main dish.

Dishes with thick creamy sauces, such as chicken korma, tikka masala or butter chicken, will be high in saturated fat and sugar, so they're best avoided if you're trying to keep your weight down. Ghee, which is clarified butter (the milk solids have been removed), is traditionally used as the base to fry Indian food. It's high in saturated fat, which adds calories but more alarmingly, a lower-cost vegetable ghee is often used that may contain harmful trans fats, due to the use of hydrogenated oils. Artificial trans fats are considered to increase the risk of heart disease, as they cannot be processed by the body and may lead to fatty deposits building up in the arteries.

On the plus side, Indian food is full of wonderful varied vegetable dishes that have much to offer in health terms. Dhal is a thick stew made with pulses such as lentils, peas or beans. These are an excellent source of soluble fibre, which can help to regulate cholesterol. Potato dishes such as sag aloo (with spinach) or aloo gobi (with cauliflower) are a good

THE RIGHT BITE

A tomato-based dish, such as Rogan Josh, is a good option as it contains less than half the saturated fat of a korma, and is far lower in calories. Choosing a vegetable side dish instead of rice or bread will keep the carb content much lower and provide the added benefits of increasing the overall fibre and antioxidant level.

way to include starch without heaping on the rice – spinach and cauliflower contain immune-boosting antioxidants.

ONE SIMPLE WAY to improve the nutritional breakdown of an Indian takeout is to prepare brown rice at home instead of ordering a portion of white rice, as it contains eight times the amount of fibre found in boiled white rice. Brown rice is also a useful source of magnesium. Optimum levels of fibre and magnesium play a key role in relieving constipation and promoting healthy digestion.

CHINESE FOOD

There is a huge variety of dishes available on a Chinese takeout menu and the nutritional value can vary from excellent to pretty scary. As with most East Asian food, the base for Chinese food usually includes ginger, garlic, chilli, spring onions/scallions and soy or fish sauce, although the proportions will vary according to the region, not to mention the international interpretations of Chinese food. These ingredients have much to recommend them, and both ginger and garlic are believed to have anti-inflammatory, antibacterial and even antioxidant properties. Ginger is also commonly used to help relieve symptoms of nausea in pregnant women.

CHINESE FOOD COMMONLY CONTAINS an additive called monosodium glutamate (MSG), used to add flavour to the sauces. Some people can be sensitive to this and experience headaches and muscle sensitivity after eating foods that contain MSG.

NUTRITION NUMBERS

↳ CHICKEN CHOP SUEY (350g)
Calories: 397 » Saturated fat: 3g
Protein: 34g » Carbohydrate: 32g
Sugars: 9g » Salt: 3g

↳ SWEET & SOUR PORK BALLS (x4)
Calories: 507 » Saturated fat: 47g
Protein: 9g » Carbohydrate: 24g
Sugars: 4g » Salt: 1g

↳ EGG FRIED RICE (100g)
Calories: 186 » Saturated fat: 1g
Protein: 4g » Carbohydrate: 33g
Sugars: 1g » Salt: 1g

↳ FRIED VEGETABLE SPRING ROLLS (per unit)
Calories: 149 » Saturated fat: 3g
Protein: 2g » Carbohydrate: 18g
Sugars: 1g » Salt: 0.5g

↳ WONTON SOUP (per 250g)
Calories: 187 » Saturated fat: 2g
Protein: 14g » Carbohydrate: 14g
Sugars: 1g » Salt: 2g

Chinese food contains a range of different fibrous vegetables with antioxidant properties and a common staple is Chinese cabbage. This is a veritable nutrition powerhouse, full of antioxidants and containing plant compounds that are considered to have powerful anti-cancer properties.

The cooking methods of Chinese food are a potential downside. You need to look out for one key word on the menu, and that is 'crispy'. Anything that's crispy is likely to be battered and deep-fried, which send the fat content and calorie count soaring. Deep-fried sweet and sour pork balls are definitely one to watch – pork is already high in saturated fat and if you take into account the batter, 4 small pork balls with a couple of spoons of egg-fried rice adds up to over 700 calories.

Eating large quantities of deep-fried food on a regular basis may result in fatty deposits in the arteries, increasing the risk of coronary heart disease. Opting for the steamed version of dumplings or spring rolls can help to significantly reduce the calorie count, as well as limiting your exposure to excessive levels of batter. A simple stir-fried meat and

THE RIGHT BITE

Avoiding deep-fried 'crispy' dishes and choosing a chop suey or similar stir-fried dish is your best bet. This means you'll be getting all the health benefits from the ginger and garlic-based sauces, while keeping the calorie and fat content to a respectable level, maintaining blood sugar levels, and limiting the exposure to potentially harmful fats. A vegetable side dish rather than rice is the best option – if you do have rice, then choose plain boiled rice. Soups are another low-calorie and low-fat option.

vegetable dish can ensure you enjoy all the potential benefits of Chinese food while avoiding the downside.

WATCH OUT FOR CALORIE-LADEN EXTRAS. If you've been tucking into a handful of prawn/shrimp crackers while you wait, then you're likely to have consumed nearly 300 calories before you even start the main meal.

Bars and Pubs

tots, shots and (salted) nots

Many people enjoy a quick tipple from time to time, on the basis that a little of what you fancy does you good, but how much is too much? The media is full of conflicting advice about the risks and benefits of alcohol so it can be difficult to know the best approach.

What is clear is that your risk of heart disease, liver disease and certain cancers increases exponentially if you're regularly exceeding the recommended weekly limits. Of course, if you're young and fit, you may think that any such risk applies to people who are older and fatter than you are, especially if you're not troubled with hangovers.

That's not the case: alcohol has a tremendously ageing impact on the body, not just on the skin but also in the strain that it puts on the body cells and systems. If that's still not enough to encourage you to consider limiting your intake, then be aware that a trip to your local bar can wreak havoc on your waistline. Alcohol can be very high in sugar, so you could easily be knocking back high levels of sugar without even realizing it.

> Alcohol has a tremendously ageing impact on the skin, body cells and systems

Regular alcohol consumption also keeps your liver very busy managing the detoxification process. That means that it doesn't have the time to focus on its many other jobs, such as energy production, fat metabolism, processing hormones, storage of vitamins A, B12, D, E and K, production of bile and capturing and digesting harmful bacteria, to name but a few. If you regularly suffer from niggling issues such as low energy, poor sleep, colds and infections, PMS or digestive discomfort, then it could be time to give your liver a break.

It's not just the alcohol that's an issue here, as most pubs and bars are well stocked with snacks that are packed with salt, refined carbohydrate and trans fats, so there are many pitfalls for the unwary. Read on to find out how you can limit the damage and even enjoy the residual health benefits of moderate alcohol consumption.

BEER

One of the challenges with beer is the sheer volume that's consumed – per 100ml it's lower in calories and alcohol content than wine, but the accumulation of several pints or bottles is where the damage can be done and the units can quickly add up to a concerning level. A 330ml bottle of extra strong lager contains about 3 units of alcohol, so enjoying what may seem like a modest 2 bottles a day adds up to a hefty 21 units of alcohol over the course of a week.

Beers, lagers, ale and stout may not taste sweet but the sugar content is still pretty significant, which can be bad news for your waistline. For those who enjoy a pint, this can rack up to 3 teaspoons of

EXCEEDING WEEKLY GUIDELINES for alcohol consumption can put you at risk of a range of chronic conditions such as heart disease, bowel cancer and fatty liver disease, not to mention more immediate concerns such as bloodshot eyes, weight gain and, for men, the infamous 'brewer's droop'.

NUTRITION NUMBERS
per pint (568ml)

↳ BITTER
Calories: 168 » Sugars: 12g
Units of alcohol: 2.3

↳ BROWN ALE
Calories: 168 » Sugars: 17g
Units of alcohol: 2.5

↳ STOUT
Calories: 168 » Sugars: 8g
Units of alcohol: 2.3

↳ LAGER
Calories: 256 » Sugars: 13g
Units of alcohol: 2.7

↳ EXTRA STRONG LAGER
(per 330ml bottle)
Calories: 244 » Sugars: 8g
Units of alcohol: 3

sugar for each pint and even the 330ml bottles contain 2 teaspoons each, so there's no escape. If you're prepared to drink low-alcohol or alcohol-free beers, these contain about half the sugar of a standard beer, as well as helping to keep you sober.

In sugar terms, there are some small differences between the different types of beer that you might want to take into account if you're watching your weight. Stout is the lowest sugar option by far, and then in close succession comes bitter, premium lager and brown ale.

In the past, stout has been recommended to pregnant women and it's still popularly believed that it has a number of health benefits, in particular that it's a good source of iron. It's true that stout is the only form of beer to contain iron, but the amount is minimal at 0.2mg per 100ml. To put this into context, a woman would have to drink 15 pints of stout per day to achieve her recommended daily allowance of iron.

It's not all bad news, though, as daily consumption of one standard 330ml bottle of lager is believed to increase antioxidant activity in the blood, boosting

THE RIGHT BITE

The smart beer drinker's choice is stout, as it's relatively lower in sugar and alcohol than other beers. Standard rather than premium lagers or bitters are a fairly safe option, but extra-strength lagers are definitely the ones to watch, with a double whammy of calories and sugar. Of course, if you're prepared to stick to one 330ml serving per day, then you can choose whichever beer you fancy.

the immune system. In this case, less is definitely more, as the same study showed that drinking three 330ml bottles of lager per day had a pro-oxidant effect, which can result in cell and tissue damage.

IF YOU'RE TRYING TO LIMIT YOUR BEER INTAKE, then take a look at the glass you're using, as it might make a difference. A recent study showed that using a tall straight glass rather than a curved glass to drink lager could slow the drinking rate by up to 60%.

WINE

When it comes to wine, much depends on your choice of colour and bubbles, as the sugar content varies dramatically according to the grape and the method used. If weight loss is your goal, don't be confused by the calories, as they're not the key thing: what you need to know is how much sugar you might be consuming.

There is a sugar pecking order, with the lowest sugar content found in red wine. After that, it goes up the ranks in this order: from dry white (such as Sauvignon Blanc), rosé and medium white wines (such as Pinot Grigio) to sparkling wines and sweet white wines (such as Sauternes), which contain up to 2 teaspoons of sugar per glass. This rather negates the popular urban myth that champagne is slimming.

THE WEEKLY GUIDELINES FOR ALCOHOL CONSUMPTION in the UK are 14 units for women and 21 units for men. The US weekly guidelines are 7 units for women and 14 units for men.

NUTRITION NUMBERS
per 175ml glass

↳ RED WINE
Calories: 133 » Sugars: 0.3g
Units of alcohol: 2.3

↳ DRY WHITE WINE
Calories: 137 » Sugars: 1g
Units of alcohol: 2.3

↳ MEDIUM WHITE WINE
Calories: 141 » Sugars: 5g
Units of alcohol: 2.3

↳ SWEET WHITE WINE
Calories: 164 » Sugars: 10g
Units of alcohol: 2.3

↳ SPARKLING WINE (125ml glass)
Calories: 89 » Sugars: 6g
Units of alcohol: 1.7

Sugar is the single biggest factor when it comes to weight gain and abdominal fat in particular. You're unlikely to achieve a six-pack or slip into your skinny jeans if you're over-indulging regularly. Just 2 small (175ml) glasses of medium white wine contain about 3 teaspoons of sugar, so if you're watching your weight it's a smart move to resist the temptation to have an extra glass.

The size of glass is important, as it makes a big difference to the number of alcohol units you consume. Enjoying two 250ml glasses over a night out may seem moderate, but it can add up to 7 units of alcohol, which is very close to the recommended limits in some countries.

It's not all bad news, however, as wine has some potential health benefits. Studies have shown that antioxidants found in red wine may have a protective effect on the heart, prevent blood clots and regulate cholesterol levels. The key here is moderation, as the studies are based on the consumption of a very small daily amount, which means you'd need to limit yourself to one small glass in order to derive the benefit. As with other types of alcohol, large quantities of wine

THE RIGHT BITE

The clear choice here is red wine as it's the lowest in sugar and has the added fringe benefits of containing some protective antioxidants. If that's really not to your taste, a white wine spritzer (with soda water, not lemonade) could be the way to go, as you can reduce the level of sugar by reducing the volume of wine.

drunk on a daily basis increases the risk of heart disease and certain cancers, so when it comes to wine, less is definitely more and spreading your allocated intake of units across the week is the way to go.

A 750ML BOTTLE OF 13.5% RED, WHITE OR ROSÉ WINE contains 10 units of alcohol. If the wine is stronger than 13.5%, then the number of units increases proportionally. Bars are now serving large 250ml glasses of wine, so you're consuming more than 3 units in just one glass.

CIDER

The alcoholic beverage cider (known in some countries as hard cider to distinguish it from non-alcoholic cider) is a fermented drink made from unfiltered apple juice. It has always been popular in the UK but has been enjoying a resurgence in popularity in recent years.

The popular phrase 'an apple a day keeps the doctor away' is more than just an old wives' tale. Apples are packed with a whole range of antioxidants such as quercetin, which is a powerful anti-inflammatory and which is believed to support heart health and protect against chronic disease. Antioxidant levels in half a pint of cider appear to be roughly similar to a glass of red wine, suggesting

HAVING A DAILY DOSE OF APPLE CIDER VINEGAR (in the raw, unfiltered form) in water is associated with a host of health benefits, such as improved digestion, speeding up the metabolism, modulating the immune system and enhancing calcium absorption.

NUTRITION NUMBERS
per pint (568ml)

↳ DRY CIDER
Calories: 201 » Sugars: 15g
Units of alcohol: 2.6

↳ SWEET CIDER
Calories: 235 » Sugars: 24g
Units of alcohol: 2.5

↳ PREMIUM CIDER / SCRUMPY
Calories: 380 » Sugars: 40
Units of alcohol: 4

that a small glass of cider each day could prove beneficial to health. A recent study has also shown that antioxidants in cider are absorbed extremely quickly into the bloodstream, enhancing the potential health benefits.

However, all forms of processing can impact on antioxidant levels. The juicing process varies according to country and manufacturer, and intensive juicing may reduce antioxidants: some studies have shown that traditional pulp and pressing methods are the least disruptive to antioxidants.

A note of caution: as with other forms of alcohol, the risks associated with regular consumption of larger quantities are likely to negate any potential antioxidant boost. Some of the premium offerings of cider are very high in alcohol, and just one pint adds up to nearly 6 units. If you're enjoying a few pints over the course of an evening, it won't be difficult to exceed the weekly recommended limit in just one go.

There is another downside to cider as it's a very sugary option – a pint of premium cider contains the equivalent of 10 teaspoons of sugar, which is three

THE RIGHT BITE

Sticking to dry cider is easily the best option, as it's the lowest in both calories and sugar. Ideally, limit yourself to just the one pint as, even with dry cider, the sugar levels can creep up to the equivalent of 10-15 teaspoons of sugar if you indulge in 3-4 pints on a night out.

times as much as a pint of premium lager. If you're regularly enjoying 4-5 pints of premium cider over the course of a week, this can quickly add up to the equivalent of the total recommended daily amount of calories, which will soon have a detrimental impact on your waistline.

IN ANTIOXIDANT TERMS, not all apples are equal, so the antioxidant content of cider will vary according to the manufacturer's choice of apple. As you're unlikely to know which apples are used, drinking vast quantities of cider is probably not the most efficient way of trying to boost antioxidant levels.

SPIRITS

Spirits have been used for centuries for various medicinal purposes and a hot toddy made with whisky or rum is still a favourite home remedy for a cold. Although there is no evidence to suggest that this can help, some symptom relief can be derived from the steam produced by the hot drink.

As with other types of alcohol, there is some evidence to suggest that moderate consumption can help reduce the risk of heart attacks by influencing the blood clotting that can commonly lead to heart attacks or strokes. The key word here is 'moderate', and relates to one small glass per day, as studies have shown that as you increase your intake to three glasses per day the risk of cardiovascular disease

ACCORDING TO A RECENT STUDY, all alcoholic drinks can change the pH of saliva, making it more acidic, which isn't great for dental health. However, only whisky can actually strip calcium from the surface of the tooth.

NUTRITION NUMBERS

↳ SPIRITS (40% e.g. vodka, whisky) per 25ml measure
Calories: 55 » Sugars: traces
Units of alcohol: 1

↳ HIGH-STRENGTH LIQUEURS (e.g. Cointreau, Pernod, Drambuie, Southern Comfort) per 50ml measure
Calories: 157 » Sugars: 12g
Units of alcohol: 1.8

↳ MEDIUM-STRENGTH LIQUEURS (e.g. cherry brandy, Tia Maria) per 50ml measure
Calories: 131 » Sugars: 16g
Units of alcohol: 1

↳ CREAM LIQUEUR (e.g. Baileys Irish Cream) per 50ml measure
Calories: 162 » Sugars: 12g
Units of alcohol: 0.8

↳ FORTIFIED WINE (e.g. medium sherry, port) per 50ml measure
Calories: 68 » Sugars: 5g
Units of alcohol: 1

increases dramatically. Training yourself to ask for a single rather than a double measure could make all the difference. If you're drinking at home, then consider investing in a spirits measure, as the 25ml measure that represents a single spirit is very hard to achieve if you're pouring with a liberal hand.

Spirits are much higher in calories than other types of alcohol, but the proportional volume means you're less likely to consume as many calories as beer or wine, especially if you stick to single measures. There's also the added advantage that the classic 40% spirits such as whisky, brandy, vodka, gin and rum contain only traces of sugar. This makes them the smart choice if weight management is your goal, especially if you choose your mixer with care.

Popular liqueurs on the other hand are a minefield for the unwary – drinks such as Cointreau, Pernod, Baileys Irish Cream, cherry brandy or Southern Comfort are packed with calories and sugar. These tend be served in 50ml measures in bars, which means you can be consuming the equivalent of up to 4 teaspoons of sugar in one small glass.

THE RIGHT BITE

Moderation is the key if you want to optimize heart health, as well as being kind to your liver. The smart choice is a single 40% spirit, and if you want to make it last a bit longer then a carefully selected mixer is the way to do it. A single measure vodka and soda would be an ideal choice – as you're avoiding both sugar and artificial sweeteners, which will help to keep the inches off your waistline.

ALCOHOL LOWERS THE BODY TEMPERATURE, so a nip of brandy on a cold day won't actually help matters. By dilating the blood vessels near the skin, blood (and heat) will move to the skin and away from your vital organs, so you need to be especially careful about walking home in freezing temperatures if you've been drinking heavily, as this can lead to hypothermia.

SOFT DRINKS

Soft drinks can be a minefield of sugar or artificial sweeteners, as well as a range of chemical additives and preservatives.

It might seem an obvious choice to opt for a diet soda, so that you can keep the sugar to a minimum, especially when you realize that a 330ml can of regular cola contains 9 teaspoons of sugar. The problem with the diet sodas starts when you look at the ingredients – the longer the list, the more processed a product it is. The jury's still out about the potential health risks of aspartame, which is the

BEWARE HIGH FRUCTOSE CORN SYRUP (HFCS) – strict quotas have been imposed in a number of countries, but in North and Latin America, and some Eastern European and Asian countries it is commonly used to sweeten popular carbonated drinks. The use of HFCS is widely considered to be contributing to a growing obesity problem, as well as being associated to an increased risk of type 2 diabetes.

NUTRITION NUMBERS

↳ REGULAR COLA (per 330ml can)
Calories: 140 » Sugars: 35g
Caffeine: 30mg

↳ CAFFEINATED ENERGY DRINK
(per 250ml can)
Calories: 150 » Sugars: 30g
Caffeine: 80mg

↳ LEMONADE (per 330ml can)
Calories: 125 » Sugars: 25g

↳ ORANGEADE (per 330ml can)
Calories: 165 » Sugars: 33g

↳ FRUIT JUICE FROM CONCENTRATE
(per 160ml bottle)
Calories: 72 » Sugars: 15g

↳ FRUIT DRINK (per 275ml)
Calories: 88 » Sugars: 20g

most common sweetener used in diet sodas, although recent studies suggest that it's safe. However, there remains a school of thought that believes that diet sodas can increase appetite, possibly by confusing the body into expecting the calorie load that would normally come with drinking something that tastes so sweet, and compensating accordingly.

If a can of cola is your preference, then you're adding phosphoric acid (which can damage tooth enamel) and about 30mg of caffeine into the mix. Popular caffeinated energy drinks contain roughly 80mg of caffeine and 4 teaspoons of sugar per 250ml can. This double whammy of sugar plus stimulant will send your blood sugar soaring, generating the insulin response which will encourage your body to store excess sugar as fat. If you use it as a mixer with alcohol, this is likely to send your blood pressure sky-high at the same time.

The other popular options tend to be fruit juices or fruit drinks. These may seem healthy but often contain added sugar, as well as natural fruit sugars. Most fruit juices in bars are concentrated, containing around 4 teaspoons of sugar.

THE RIGHT BITE

Sparkling water with a slice of lemon is a great option here – no sugar, no additives and no preservatives as well as the added bonus of helping to avoid peer pressure, as you can pretend it's a gin and tonic. Adding a dash of cordial, such as lime or elderflower, can liven it up without doing too much damage. You could also consider a tomato juice, as it contains less than half the calories and sugar content of a fruit juice.

Fruit drinks commonly contain even more sugar, as well as sweeteners and a range of additives, preservatives and flavourings, and very little genuine fruit.

WATCH OUT FOR YOUR CAFFEINE LEVELS if you're drinking a lot of caffeinated sodas during the day, on top of tea and coffee. You could easily be exceeding the recommended daily limit of 400mg, which will have a hugely disruptive impact on your sleep.

NUTS

If only food manufacturers hadn't added salt to the more popular nuts, they would be an overall winner of a snack. They're an excellent source of plant protein, which helps to promote sustained energy and smooth muscle tone. They're also packed with unsaturated fats, fibre and some key vitamins and minerals. The downside is that 100g of salted nuts contains around 2g of salt, a third of the guideline daily allowance, so beware if you have been told to regulate salt intake.

Not all nuts are equal, and a smart choice, depending on what's available, could directly support your

BOTH OMEGA 3 AND OMEGA 6 FATTY ACIDS are key to optimal health, but the ratio is key as excessive levels of omega 6 can cause inflammation and may increase the risk of chronic disease. High levels of palm oil in the modern diet have disrupted this ratio, so choosing nuts that are rich in omega 3 can help redress the balance.

NUTRITION NUMBERS
per 100g roasted, salted nuts

↳ ALMONDS
Calories: 612 » Protein: 21g
Fibre: 7g » Saturated fat: 4g
Monounsaturated fat: 38g
Salt: 1g

↳ CASHEWS
Calories: 611 » Protein: 20g
Fibre: 3g » Saturated fat: 10g
Monounsaturated fat: 29g
Salt: 1g

↳ PEANUTS
Calories: 589 » Protein: 25g
Fibre: 6g » Saturated fat: 9g
Monounsaturated fat: 22g
Salt: 2g

↳ PISTACHIOS
Calories: 601 » Protein: 18g
Fibre: 6g » Saturated fat: 7g
Monounsaturated fat: 18g
Salt: 1.3g

health goals. Almonds are very high in monounsaturated fatty acids, and studies have shown that daily consumption of almonds can help to reduce levels of bad LDL cholesterol. Eating whole almonds with their skins on exposes you to a range of antioxidants, which help to reduce the risk of heart disease and they also help to regulate blood sugar levels. Don't neglect Brazil nuts and walnuts; they're full of omega 3, which helps to reduce inflammation and the build-up of plaque in the blood vessels, stabilize heart rhythms and improve blood flow.

Peanuts and cashews are actually legumes and not nuts at all and they contain more starch than traditional nuts, so that they are more likely to lead to weight gain. Cashews are particularly starchy, containing over four times as much starch as an almond and double the starch of a peanut. The fat profile is also different, being generally higher in saturated fats than other nuts.

When it comes to micronutrients, there's more good news: both pistachios and almonds are full of potassium for a healthy heart and an excellent source of folate and vitamin E, both of which play

a key role in fertility. Cashews are rich in zinc, which is important for almost every bodily system, including the brain and nervous system, reproduction, energy, the immune system and great skin and hair. Peanuts are a good source of B vitamins, which are vital for energy production, as well as calming the nervous system.

THE RIGHT BITE

Raw, unsalted nuts (if available) are definitely the ones to choose, as roasting nuts reduces the nutrient content and eating salted nuts can easily take you over the daily recommended limit for salt. The best nuts to choose are almonds – they're practically a 'superfood'.

REMEMBER, HEALTHY EATING IS NOT ABOUT THE CALORIES. But if you still can't bring yourself to eat nuts because you think they're fattening, then it might help to know that essential fatty acids help to speed up the metabolism and burn fat.

POTATO CHIPS

Crisps and other potato chips are the single most common snack found in bars, partly because the high salt content helps you to work up a thirst and sends you back to the bar for another drink – good news for the landlord's profits. They're not so good for your health, though – they might be tasty but they're not nutritious: they are highly processed and essentially a blend of fat and sugar, due to the high levels of potato starch.

This combination of fat, sugar and salt is problematic, as these are the foods that we instinctively crave and the more

POTATO CHIPS COMMONLY CONTAIN ACRYLAMIDE, which is a chemical produced by frying starch at very high temperatures. A 2009 study showed that daily intake of acrylamide through eating large amounts of potato chips causes increased levels of C-reactive protein, which is an inflammatory marker considered to be a risk factor for heart disease.

NUTRITION NUMBERS
per 100g

↳ POTATO CHIPS
Calories: 530 » Carbohydrate: 53g
Fat: 34g » Salt: 2g » Fibre: 5g

↳ ROOT VEGETABLE CRISPS
Calories: 515 » Carbohydrate: 42g
Fat: 33g » Salt: 0.8g » Fibre: 11g

↳ TORTILLA CHIPS
Calories: 459 » Carbohydrate: 60g
Fat: 23g » Salt: 2g » Fibre: 5g

you eat of them the more you're likely to want. Studies have shown that this type of manufactured snack has a much more dramatic impact on blood glucose levels than a wholefood snack, generating a more immediate insulin response. Regular consumption of these energy-dense snacks may also disrupt the body's satiety response, which is the mechanism that tells you when you're full. Both of these issues will have a direct impact on your weight: the insulin response encourages your body to store excess sugar as fat and an impaired satiety response will result in poor portion control and overeating.

There's also the salt content to consider, as this can vary dramatically according to the brand. It averages at about 0.5g, but can be as much as 1g per small 25g packet, and if the chips are served in a bowl, you're likely to be eating a lot more than a 25g packet, without even realizing. Daily guidelines advise a maximum of 6g of salt per day and it's easy to achieve this even if you don't add salt to your food, as processed foods, bread, breakfast cereals and ready-meals tend to contain a healthy dose. Excessive

THE RIGHT BITE

If root vegetable crisps are available, they are a marginally better option. Although the fat and starch levels are roughly similar, they contain twice as much fibre and half the amount of salt of standard crisps or potato chips. The fibre will keep you going for longer and reduce the possibility of a rapid insulin response and the subsequent blood sugar crash that leads to sugar and carb cravings. If not, then nuts are a much better option than crisps, as they contain distinctly more nutritional value.

salt levels can result in high blood pressure, increasing the risk of heart disease and strokes, and water retention, resulting in bloating and swelling.

IF YOU HAVE A STANDARD 25G PACKET OF POTATO CHIPS EVERY DAY, then you're consuming around 3,000g of fat per year with just one daily snack.

Picnics

breads, spreads and
other dreads

With the arrival of summer, heading outdoors to enjoy a picnic is a must in order to make the most of the good weather. Picnics are a wonderful opportunity to tuck into a range of finger food and snacks and eating outdoors tends to stimulate the appetite, so that it could be easy to overdo things. Traditional picnics can wreak havoc on a careful diet, but there are lots of ways around this and some simple opportunities to pick up a quick win on the health front.

As with so many dining contexts, it's only too easy to overdo the refined carbohydrate that has a direct impact on your waistline, as well as robbing you of the rich nutrient profile found in the wholegrain. A careful choice of bread or pastry can make all the difference to both your waistline and your wellbeing. In this chapter, we'll examine the various options available and guide you through the minefield of starch that the picnic can become so that you don't end up feeling bloated and uncomfortable.

Avoid a minefield of starch that can leave you feeling bloated and uncomfortable

With a picnic, fatty meats and snacks are often on the menu so it's easy to fall into the habit of tucking into the types of food that you'd normally avoid because they're processed. As in so many cases, a little of what you fancy won't do you too much harm, so portion control is the order of the day with some of the more indulgent offerings and a focus on protein-rich snacks featuring eggs, houmous, lean meat or fish can help to make sure you don't overdo things.

Picking one or two indulgences and playing it safe with the other foods is one way to make sure that you're able to avoid being a party pooper, while ensuring that you limit the damage and optimize the potential health benefits. And there are quite a few – houmous, guacamole, soft cheese, focaccia and tomato tarts to name but a few. Read on to find out how to transform your picnics into a nutritional powerhouse.

QUICHES & TARTS

Most quiches contain a mixture of eggs, cream or milk and cheese, which has immediate implications in terms of fat content. Tarts are more likely to contain one or more vegetables without the binding egg mixture of a quiche, which is why home-made tarts with soft vegetables such as onion or tomato can work so well. The protein content of a vegetable tart will be low and so it is less likely to keep you going than a protein-rich quiche, but as it also contains roughly half the fat content, there is much to recommend it.

QUICHES OR TARTS WITH ONIONS OR LEEKS are an excellent option for digestive health. These are part of the allium family, which includes garlic and chives. Allium vegetables contain inulin, a non-digestible form of fibre that stimulates the growth of beneficial bacteria in the gut.

NUTRITION NUMBERS
per 150g slice

↳ QUICHE LORRAINE
Calories: 412 » Carbohydrate: 20g
Sugars: 3g » Total fat: 28g
Saturated fat: 14g » Protein: 18g

↳ ROASTED VEGETABLE TART
Calories: 302 » Carbohydrate: 32g
Sugars: 8g » Total fat: 16g
Saturated fat: 6g » Protein: 4g

↳ CHEESE & ONION TART
Calories: 492 » Carbohydrate: 35g
Sugars: 5g » Total fat:33g
Saturated fat: 14g » Protein: 13g

↳ SMOKED SALMON & SPINACH QUICHE
Calories: 433 » Carbohydrate: 26g
Sugars: 3g » Total fat: 30g
Saturated fat: 12g » Protein: 13g

A home-made quiche is preferable as you will avoid the additives and preservatives used to increase the shelf life of a commercially made quiche. A large quiche contains roughly 5 eggs, so even one slice will pack a powerful protein punch. Protein plays a key part in growth and repair of cells and is very important for optimal energy levels, as well as ensuring healthy nails and hair. Despite a bad press in recent years, eggs are practically a superfood and research has consistently shown that while they may contain dietary cholesterol, this does not impact on the levels of bad LDL cholesterol that is currently believed to be a risk factor for cardiovascular disease.

Choose a quiche or tart carefully to optimize the potential health benefits. Steering clear of a classic Quiche Lorraine could be wise, as bacon is highly processed and very salty, a combination that can adversely affect heart health and blood pressure levels. However, quiches that contain green vegetables, such as broccoli or spinach, expose you to a range of protective antioxidants, boosting the micronutrient value and increasing fibre levels to support a healthy digestion.

THE RIGHT BITE

A vegetable-rich quiche is the best option, as this avoids the processed bacon found in the classic Quiche Lorraine and allows you to benefit from the residual health benefits of mixing eggs with vegetables – a classic protein-fibre blend.

Limiting the amount of pastry and just tucking into the filling will significantly reduce the carb levels, which is much kinder to the waistline. Although not technically a quiche, a vegetable frittata is worth consideration – this has the dual advantage of losing the starchy carbohydrate pastry and the fatty cream while retaining the benefits of the eggs.

A TOMATO TART HAS A HIDDEN BONUS, as cooked tomatoes contain higher levels of lycopene than raw tomatoes. Lycopene is a powerful antioxidant that plays a key part in male health and can help to reduce the risk of prostate cancer.

PIES, PASTIES & SAUSAGE ROLLS

Pies, pasties and sausage rolls are high in calories and starchy carbohydrate and will be no friend to your waistline. Home-made products have a clear advantage, as you can control the quality of the ingredients – using sausage meat with more than 80% pork content or locally produced organic beef, for example, means that you're avoiding exposure to the additives, preservatives and toxins that may be present in processed forms of the product. Wholemeal pastry boosts

LIMITING YOURSELF TO JUST TWO SAUSAGE ROLLS may seem like a moderate approach but it adds up to over 400 calories and 10g of saturated fat, which is half the recommended daily intake, as well as containing a hefty dose of salt. If heart health is a concern, this is one to avoid.

NUTRITION NUMBERS

↳ PORK PIE
(per 100g individual small pie)
Calories: 379 » Protein: 10g
Carbohydrate: 26g » Sugars: 1.5g
Fibre: 3g » Total fat: 26g
Saturated fat: 10g » Salt: 1.5g

↳ SAUSAGE ROLL
(per 60g individual serving)
Calories: 208 » Protein: 5g
Carbohydrate: 16g » Sugars: 1g
Fibre: 2g » Total fat: 13g
Saturated fat: 5g » Salt: 1g

↳ CORNISH PASTY
(per medium-size 200g pasty)
Calories: 556 » Protein: 16g
Carbohydrate: 48g » Sugars: 4g
Fibre: 6g » Total fat: 34g
Saturated fat: 16g » Salt: 1g

↳ VEGETABLE PASTY
(per medium-size 200g pasty)
Calories: 588 » Protein: 8g
Carbohydrate: 60g » Sugars: 3g
Fibre: 7g » Total fat: 34g
Saturated fat: 12g » Salt: 0.3g

the fibre content of the product and reduces levels of refined carbohydrate.

In principle, a fresh Cornish pasty made with a filling of lean beef, potato, swede/rutabaga or turnip and onion has much to recommend it, as it contains a blend of lean protein and fibrous vegetables that help to maintain blood sugar levels. Home-made pork pie is usually made with a mixture of pork belly and shoulder, and while pork is quite a fatty meat, it is also an excellent source of protein, iron and B vitamins, which are vital for energy. Even a home-made sausage roll can be a simple snack of sausage meat and pastry, which will never be a low-calorie option, but needn't necessarily be a health risk when eaten in moderation.

However, when these products are produced in bulk by food manufacturers, other considerations, such as shelf life, come into play and it's important to look at the label closely. Processed meat remains under scrutiny as there is an association with the increased risk of chronic disease when eaten regularly and in large quantities. The longer the ingredients list, the more processed the product. Any general references to

THE RIGHT BITE

If it's possible to enjoy a home-made product, then you'll straight away be limiting the potential damage in health terms. If not, check the label of commercial products and opt for the product that has the fewest and simplest ingredients, as this is likely to reduce your exposure to artificial preservatives. A wholemeal pasty with lean meat and a blend of vegetables is likely to be your best bet – cutting it in half can help keep the numbers down in terms of calorie, fat and salt content.

preservatives is likely to mean nitrites have been used to preserve the meat and maintain the pink colour that's so characteristic of pork pie, for example.

STUDIES SUGGEST THAT CONSUMING PROCESSED MEATS in the form of commercial pies and pasties on a regular basis may increase the risk of chronic disease, so enjoying these foods strictly in moderation is the key.

BREAD

White bread has a poorer nutritional profile than wholemeal bread as the refining process removes the bran and the germ, which are the most nutritious parts. Wholemeal breads are a natural source of B vitamins that support the nervous system and play a key role in energy production. They also contain vitamin E, an antioxidant that may play a part in reducing the risk of coronary heart disease as well as supporting eye health and protecting against macular degeneration.

White bread has a high glycaemic index, which can result in a blood sugar spike and lead to weight gain. By opting

WHOLEMEAL BREAD CONTAINS HIGH LEVELS OF PHYTIC ACID, which can block the absorption of key minerals such as zinc and iron. Opting for breads made with spelt, which is a more ancient form of grain and generally far less processed, can help reduce exposure to these phytates.

NUTRITION NUMBERS

↳ FRENCH STICK (per 80g portion)
Calories: 210 » Carbohydrate: 44g
Sugars: 2g » Fibre: 2g

↳ FOCACCIA (per 80g portion)
Calories: 237 » Carbohydrate: 36g
Sugars: 1g » Fibre: 2g

↳ CIABATTA (per roll)
Calories: 208 » Carbohydrate: 36g
Sugars: 2g » Fibre: 2g

↳ SOFT WHITE ROLL (per unit)
Calories: 203 » Carbohydrate: 41g
Sugars: 2g » Fibre: 2g

↳ WHOLEMEAL ROLL (per unit)
Calories: 195 » Carbohydrate: 37g
Sugars: 2g » Fibre: 4g

↳ MULTIGRAIN ROLL (per unit)
Calories: 207 » Carbohydrate: 34g
Sugars: 3g » Fibre: 4g

↳ WHITE SOURDOUGH (per 80g)
Calories: 174 » Carbohydrate: 36g
Sugars: 1g » Fibre: 1g

for wholemeal, the fibre content is roughly doubled, helping to maintain steady blood sugar levels, promote sustained energy and reduce sugar cravings.

Multigrain bread contains small quantities of seeds such as flax, poppy and sunflower seeds, which have many health benefits. These are excellent sources of fibre and protein and full of omega 3, which has anti-inflammatory properties, helps to protect against heart disease and supports the nervous system. Flaxseed is a good source of lignans, plant compounds with hormone-balancing properties.

More exotic offerings such as herby focaccia with rosemary or thyme can pack a powerful health punch. Rosemary contains compounds that can help to relieve inflammation of the airways in conditions such as asthma; thyme oils are believed to have antimicrobial properties that can help to protect against a range of bacterial or fungal infection.

A note of caution – high levels of wheat can irritate a sensitive digestion, especially during times of stress. Keeping it to a minimum or replacing it with rye or spelt may help to reduce bloating.

THE RIGHT BITE

A wholemeal version of the bread of your choice will double the fibre content and ensure that you benefit from the full vitamin content of the germ and all the residual health benefits. If bread tends to make you bloated, then a wholemeal sourdough, rye or spelt loaf is the one for you. A multigrain or seeded roll exposes you to a range of supportive nutrients, although you'd need to eat one on a regular basis to derive sustained health benefits.

THE NATURAL BACTERIA IN SOURDOUGH BREADS may enhance the absorption of vitamins and minerals in the flour and there is growing evidence to suggest that the gluten in sourdough may be easier to digest than in other breads, which makes it an interesting option for people who struggle with a gluten or wheat sensitivity.

CHEESE

Cheese is made up of protein and fat in roughly equal parts, depending on the type of cheese. Derived from milk, it's a natural source of calcium, which is important for bone health and muscle function, including optimal function of the heart muscle. Calcium levels are significantly higher in harder cheeses such as Cheddar or Edam, compared to softer cheeses such as brie or mozzarella.

A large proportion of the fat content of cheese is saturated fat and just an average 50g slice of Cheddar or blue cheese adds up to nearly half the daily recommended intake for women. However, despite its reputation, saturated fat is not all bad, and it plays a key role in vital functions such as the production of sex hormones and the absorption of

AS CHEESES AGE, they can develop high levels of amines, such as tyramine and tryptamine, which are by-products of protein and can trigger migraines in people who are sensitive to dietary amines.

NUTRITION NUMBERS
per 50g serving (full-fat)

↳ CHEDDAR
Calories: 208 » Protein: 13g
Total fat: 17g » Saturated fat: 11g

↳ MONTEREY JACK
Calories: 175 » Protein: 12g
Total fat: 6g » Saturated fat: 7g

↳ BRIE
Calories: 171 » Protein: 10g
Total fat: 15g » Saturated fat: 9g

↳ BLUE CHEESE
Calories: 188 » Protein: 14g
Total fat: 16g » Saturated fat: 11g

↳ HALLOUMI
Calories: 156 » Protein: 12g
Total fat: 12g » Saturated fat: 8g

↳ MOZZARELLA
Calories: 128 » Protein: 9g
Total fat: 10g » Saturated fat: 3g

vitamin D in the body, which means that stripping it out of the diet altogether may not be a smart move.

Although they may be lower in calories, processed cheese slices are far less nutrient-dense than other forms of cheese. The addition of water, whey powder, emulsifiers and preservatives means there is very little that is natural about these products and their health contribution is minimal.

Despite the ongoing trend toward eating low-fat cheese, not only does full-fat cheese have more flavour, it also exposes you to greater health benefits than the low-fat versions. Whole milk cheese contains greater proportions of omega 3 essential fatty acids, as there is a tendency for manufacturers to strip out all forms of fat when developing low-fat varieties of cheese. Full-fat varieties have the added bonus of being a valuable source of vitamins A, D, E and K, which support the immune function and promote bone heath, antioxidant minerals such as selenium and zinc, and energy-boosting iron and B vitamins.

If salt levels are a concern, it's worth noting that low-fat cheeses tend to

THE RIGHT BITE

Opt for a full-fat unprocessed cheese if you wish to optimize the health benefits. Softer cheeses are generally lower in saturated fat, if this is a concern, while harder cheeses are richer in calcium, so the choice is yours. Avoiding the saltier cheeses such as halloumi and blue cheese is worth considering if blood pressure levels need to be regulated.

contain higher levels of salt to enhance the flavour that has been stripped out with the fat. However, of all the cheeses, halloumi is by far the most salty, containing more than double the sodium content of all the other cheeses.

RECENT STUDIES SUGGEST THAT SMALL AMOUNTS OF CHEESE (25g or less) every day can help to regulate blood sugar levels and may even reduce the risk of type 2 diabetes.

SALAMI & CURED MEATS

Curing meat is a form of preservation that usually involves the addition of salt and preservatives in the form of nitrates and nitrites, or occasionally the smoking or drying of meat. Some of these techniques date back centuries, but in recent times the curing process has become more industrialized, involving the addition of chemical preservatives such as sodium nitrite, which helps the meat to retain its characteristic pink or red colour.

Cured meats such as salami or chorizo will soon add up to a fairly hefty calorie count, as a few small round slices

IF YOU'RE A MIGRAINE SUFFERER, then it may be wise to keep processed meats to a minimum. Although there is no definitive evidence-base to confirm this, it is thought that exposure to nitrates found in processed meat may trigger migraines.

NUTRITION NUMBERS

↳ SALAMI (per 30g, 4-5 slices)
Calories: 119 » Protein: 0.3g
Total fat: 10g » Saturated fat: 4g
Salt: 1.5g

↳ PARMA HAM/PROSCIUTTO (per slice)
Calories: 34 » Protein: 4g
Total fat: 2g » Saturated fat: 1g
Salt: 0.7g

↳ CHORIZO (per 30g, 4-5 slices)
Calories: 127 » Protein: 8g
Total fat: 10g » Saturated fat: 4g
Salt: 1.5g

↳ SMOKED HAM (per slice)
Calories: 25 » Protein: 4g
Total fat: 0.5g » Saturated fat: 0.2g
Salt: 0.5g

can pack in quite a few calories, largely due to the high levels of fat. Excessive consumption of processed meat is considered to increase the risk factor for contracting chronic conditions such as cardiovascular disease and some cancers.

Parma ham or prosciutto are dry-cured hams, which are usually served raw and in very thin slices. Eaten sparingly, they can be significantly lower in both calories and fat than other cured meats. However, the curing process does involve large amounts of salt – it's easy to tuck into four or five slices as the ham is cut so thinly, which can soon bring you well over half the daily recommended limit of salt. If blood pressure levels are a concern, then these are foods to enjoy in moderation.

Smoked ham may taste delicious, as the process adds a lovely woody flavour, but large amounts of salt are involved in the production. Depending on the process, smoked meat may be exposed to polycyclic aromatic hydrocarbons, toxic compounds that have been associated with increased risk of some cancers.

Chorizo can vary in quality, but at its best it is a blend of lean pork loin with

THE RIGHT BITE

With cured meats, less is definitely more. The heavily processed nature of these foods means that it's best not to consume them in excess. However, if you do want to indulge occasionally, avoid smoked meats and opt for a small portion of Parma ham.

pork belly and a good source of protein. The characteristic flavour is created by the use of pimentón, a type of smoked paprika. Paprika contains comparatively high levels of antioxidant vitamins A and C and it has historically been used as an anti-bacterial and to reduce inflammation.

IT'S UNUSUAL TO HAVE A DEFICIENCY IN SALT, as it's added to so many products, such as processed meats, breakfast cereals and bread. However, as sodium works with potassium to regulate muscle contraction, a deficiency can lead to painful cramps in certain groups of muscles.

PÂTÉS & DIPS

Pâté is essentially a blend of cooked ground meat commonly mixed with vegetables, herbs and spices to form a spreadable paste. Home-made pâté has much to recommend it, as you'll know exactly which ingredients you've used, but some commercial pâté can be extremely processed. Cheaper pâté is often made with reclaimed meat (scraps of meat blasted off the carcass with a jet, once the principal cuts have been used) and can be high in salt, saturated fat and all manner of preservatives, so that there's very little in the way of really good nutrients.

A fish pâté, such as mackerel or salmon, may be high in fat, but a large proportion is made up of heart-healthy

IF YOU SUFFER FROM GOUT, which is becoming increasingly common, tucking into mackerel pâté or taramasalata is to be avoided. Oily fish such as mackerel, fish roe and shellfish are all high in purines, which can trigger a gouty episode.

NUTRITION NUMBERS
per 50g serving

↳ SMOOTH LIVER PÂTÉ
Calories: 174 » Protein: 6g
Carbohydrate: 1g » Sugars: 0.2g
Total fat: 16g » Saturated fat: 5g
Salt: 1g

↳ MACKEREL PÂTÉ
Calories: 158 » Protein: 6g
Carbohydrate: 1g » Sugars: 0.1g
Total fat: 14g » Saturated fat: 6g
Salt: 0.5g

↳ HOUMOUS
Calories: 153 » Protein: 4g
Carbohydrate: 5g » Sugars: 0.3g
Total fat: 13g » Saturated fat: 1g
Salt: 0.5g

↳ GUACAMOLE
Calories: 98 » Protein: 0.5g
Carbohydrate: 4g » Sugars: 3g
Total fat: 9g » Saturated fat: 3g
Salt: 0.2g

omega 3 fatty acids, as well as being a great source of lean protein, iron, B vitamins, and even some vitamin D. It's also extremely simple to make, so that you can control the proportion of fish against the soft cheese, ensuring a bias in favour of polyunsaturates.

With dips, the trick is to opt for something that is nutrient-dense so that it offers a broad range of health benefits. Houmous is a much better option than sour cream and chives, even though the calorie count is similar. Houmous mostly consists of chickpeas, which are packed with protein and fibre, so it's the ideal snack to balance blood sugar and it's a good source of healthy mono- and polyunsaturated fats that play a key part in heart, hormone and brain health.

Both guacamole and taramasalata are relatively low in protein but they're good sources of mono- and polyunsaturates, which can help to reduce inflammation. If you're making your own guacamole, be generous with the avocado, as it contains extremely high levels of antioxidant carotenoids, which help to neutralize free radicals in the body that increase the risk of chronic diseases such as cancer.

THE RIGHT BITE

Houmous is the obvious winner here as the protein-fibre blend ticks all the boxes in terms of blood sugar balance, sustained energy and weight management, as well as exposing you to the highly beneficial nutrients found in chickpeas. If you eat it with chopped carrots, cucumber or cherry tomatoes, rather than breadsticks or potato chips, you'll be keeping starch to a minimum and deriving extra fibre and antioxidants from the vegetables, as well as being kind to your waistline.

CHICKPEAS ARE A NUTRITIONAL POWERHOUSE: as well as being rich in protein and essential fatty acids, they're an excellent source of fibre, which supports digestive health and regular bowel movements. The soluble fibre they contain helps to regulate cholesterol levels and they also contain plant compounds held to have hormone-balancing properties.

Barbecues

what's charred and what's barred

Freshly cooked meat with a range of salads eaten in the fresh air – what could be healthier? With the arrival of summer, the temptation to fire up the barbecue is strong and on the face of it, a barbecue ticks a lot of health boxes compared to wintertime dining options, which so often rely on unhealthy 'comfort food'.

However, there are some pitfalls to be aware of. Firstly, the cooking method itself can be problematic: cooking meat at extremely high temperatures, especially when an open flame is involved, can lead to the creation of powerful toxins that have been associated with the risk of developing some cancers. Find out more in the Meat section of this chapter along with some strategies to avoid this.

Although fish, seafood and vegetables can all feature on the barbecue, the activity mostly centres around meat in its different forms, and the quality of meat on offer makes a significant difference to the potential health benefits. Opting for lean cuts, organic and/or locally produced meat will help to avoid exposure to excessive levels of saturated fat, and artificial additives and preservatives commonly used in processed meat products, such as sausages.

It's important to pay attention to the accompaniments, as some damage can be done here, with big portions of starch in the form of bread, potato or rice. Barbecue sauce, sugary marinades and salad dressings also need to be treated with caution, as they can be relatively high in empty calories, especially if you're applying them with a liberal hand.

On the plus side, piling some quality cuts of meat or fish onto your plate along with a range of grilled vegetables and/or salad provides a nicely balanced meal that will ensure sustained energy, support digestion and expose you to a range of protective antioxidants.

> Cooking meat over an open flame can lead to the creation of powerful toxins

SAUSAGES

The first thing to look for in a sausage is the percentage of meat as this is a key factor in a good-quality sausage. Regulations will vary from country to country, but the minimum amount of pork in a pork sausage can be as low as 42%. For a chipolata, the meat content can drop as low as 32% and with other meats it may only be 30%. In all cases, this figure can include both fat and connective tissue. That leaves an awful lot of room for fillers, and poor-quality sausages are commonly bulked up with a generous blend of rusk and water. If a sausage is leaking water or white liquid into the pan,

SPICY MERGUEZ ARE MIXED WITH CUMIN AND CHILLI, which boosts the health profile of these sausages. Cumin seeds are an excellent source of iron and can help to stimulate the digestive process. Red chilli is packed with the antioxidants vitamin C and beta carotene that can have a powerfully protective effect against chronic disease.

NUTRITION NUMBERS
per sausage

↳ PORK CHIPOLATA
Calories: 65 » Protein: 4g
Total fat: 4g » Saturated fat: 2g
Carbohydrate: 2g » Salt: 0.2g

↳ VENISON SAUSAGE
Calories: 175 » Protein: 15g
Total fat: 11g » Saturated fat: 5g
Carbohydrate: 2g » Salt: 0.5g

↳ MERGUEZ SAUSAGE
Calories: 198 » Protein: 11g
Total fat: 16g » Saturated fat: 7g
Carbohydrate: 1g » Salt: 1.5g

↳ CUMBERLAND PORK SAUSAGE
Calories: 141 » Protein: 17g
Total fat: 19g » Saturated fat: 7g
Carbohydrate: 8g » Salt: 0.8g

it's a real giveaway that the ratio of filler to actual meat is pretty high.

A sausage that contains 85–90% meat is a different matter. Premium sausages tend to be far superior as there is less room for additives and preservatives as well as the benefit of the high nutrient content of fresh, quality meat. While pork is quite a fatty meat, the fat profile is a blend of saturated and monounsaturated fat in the form of oleic acid, which is considered to help protect against heart disease. It's also an excellent source of protein. Like all meats, pork is rich in vitamins B1, B6 and B12, which support energy levels and play a key part in the optimal function of the nervous system.

Venison sausages are an especially healthy option, as venison is higher in protein than other red meats, as well as containing even more iron than lamb or beef, making it an excellent energy-boosting option and helping to reduce the risk of anaemia.

Although the numbers may make chipolatas look the most attractive option, they are significantly smaller than standard sausages. However, per 100g,

THE RIGHT BITE

Opt for sausages with a high meat content and you're more likely to limit your exposure to both the connective tissue and the preservative-rich fillers that tend to be found in low-grade sausages. Aim for a minimum of 80% meat content. For added residual health benefits, an iron-rich venison sausage or a spicy merguez with antioxidants would be a great choice.

the nutritional profile is similar to other sausages, so any benefit will only be derived with minimal portions.

ALL SAUSAGES CONTAIN SOME DEGREE OF PRESERVATIVES and these can range from artificial colourings such as nitrates, to preserve the pink colour of the meat, to chemicals to enhance flavours, and polyphosphates to bind the sausage together and extend shelf life. The longer the list of ingredients, the greater the risk of artificial ingredients and chemicals.

MEAT

A growing body of research suggests there is a health risk associated with grilling meat over an open flame. This is due to the formation of two substances that have been linked to the development of cancer in animal studies: heterocyclic amines (HCAs) and polycyclic aromatic hydrocarbons (PAHs). HCAs are formed when the amino acids that make up the protein of the meat, sugars and creatine react to the very high temperature of the barbecue. PAHs form when fat from the meat drops onto the fire, causing flames generating PAHs, which then stick to the surface of the meat. PAHs may also be formed during the smoking process of meat.

While the definitive conclusions have yet to be drawn, it seems wise to limit

CHOOSE YOUR ACCOMPANYING SAUCE or marinade with care. Sugary glazes and sauces can contain the equivalent of up to 4 teaspoons of sugar per average 37ml serving, adding empty calories.

NUTRITION NUMBERS
(values when barbecued, excluding sauces or marinades)

↳ PORK SPARE RIBS (per 4 ribs)
Calories: 281 » Protein: 26g
Total fat: 17g » Saturated fat: 6g

↳ SKINLESS CHICKEN BREAST (per 150g)
Calories: 222 » Protein: 48g
Total fat: 3g » Saturated fat: 1g

↳ LEAN RUMP STEAK (per 300g)
Calories: 522 » Protein: 93g
Total fat: 17g » Saturated fat: 7g

↳ PULLED PORK SHOULDER (per 300g)
Calories: 497 » Protein: 91g
Total fat: 22g » Saturated fat: 12g

↳ BEEF BURGER (per 100g burger)
Calories: 249 » Protein: 24g
Total fat: 16g » Saturated fat: 7g

exposure to HCAs and PAHs. One way of doing this is to use lean cuts of meat, such as chicken breast, and ensure that red meat is trimmed of all fat, as this can help to avoid fat dripping onto the fire. Partially pre-cooking the meat in a microwave reduces cooking time, so the exposure to the open flame is minimal. Using smaller cuts of meat that cook more quickly, turning it regularly and discarding any charred parts of the meat may all help to reduce exposure to HCAs and PAHs.

All meat is an excellent source of protein, which is vital for the growth and repair of body cells; it also plays a key role in maintaining sustained energy levels, as it helps to ensure satiety (feeling full) after a meal. Fat levels can vary considerably: chicken and other poultry is much lower in fat than red meat. Pork is the one to watch if you are concerned about saturated fat, as it tends to be much higher per 100g than other red meats.

Of all the typical barbecued meats, iron-rich beef is the best one to opt for if you're feeling low in energy. It's also a good source of vitamin B12, which is commonly depleted in elderly people and also in those exposed to chronic stress. A deficiency in B12 results in a condition called pernicious anaemia causing extreme tiredness.

THE RIGHT BITE

The trick is to ensure that your chosen meat is as lean as possible and the fat has been trimmed off to limit the potential for harmful toxins to develop during the barbecue process. Smaller cuts will not only keep calories down, but may help to avoid the development of HCAs. An unsweetened chilli sauce is likely to be the best accompaniment as it's far lower in sugar than the average barbecue sauces.

LAMB IS AN EXCELLENT SOURCE OF ZINC, which plays a key role in a whole range of bodily systems, including the immune system, reproductive system, bone health, healthy skin and hair and the optimal function of the sense of taste and smell.

SKEWERS

The advantage of skewers on the barbecue is that it gives you the chance to mix it up a bit, interspersing the meat, fish or cheese with vegetables. This gives a much-needed fibre boost to what can be a protein and fat-heavy meal, as well as exposing you to a range of vitamins and minerals.

The meat portion on a skewer tends to be smaller than other options on the barbecue, which is one way to keep the calorie count down. Barbecuing with skewers also gives the opportunity to use seafood such as prawns/shrimp or calamari, which are excellent low-fat sources of protein, with the added benefit of polyunsaturated fats, which

THERE IS AN INCREASING AMOUNT OF RESEARCH into the therapeutic value of mushrooms, in particular with regard to modulating the actions of the immune system, relieving chronic inflammation and supporting cardiovascular health by improving circulation.

NUTRITION NUMBERS

↳ KING PRAWNS/JUMBO SHRIMP (x4)
Calories: 102 » Protein: 24g
Total fat: 0.6g » Saturated fat: 0.1g
Salt: 1g

↳ CALAMARI (unbattered, per 150g)
Calories: 138 » Protein: 29g
Total fat: 1.5g » Saturated fat: 0.3g
Salt: 0.01g

↳ CHICKEN BREAST (per 150g)
Calories: 221 » Protein: 47g
Total fat: 3g » Saturated fat: 1g
Salt: 0.2g

↳ HALLOUMI (per 150g)
Calories: 469 » Protein: 36g
Total fat: 35g » Saturated fat: 24g
Salt: 2g

↳ LAMB KOFTA (x4 meatballs)
Calories: 155 » Protein: 26g
Total fat: 13g » Saturated fat: 6g
Salt: 1g

are especially high in calamari. Seafood is also one of the rare dietary sources of iodine, which is vital for healthy thyroid function.

A halloumi skewer may seem like a healthy vegetarian option, but it's extremely high in saturated fat and salt, and is one to watch for people who have high blood pressure and are keen to manage heart health.

Loading your skewer with vegetables, such as aubergine/eggplant, onion, cherry tomatoes, mushrooms, and peppers, can add a range of health benefits. Aubergines/eggplants may not look very interesting but they contain a number of plant compounds such as nasunin, an antioxidant that may help to reduce the growth of cancer cells and chlorogenic acid, which is believed to play a part in regulating cholesterol levels. Red peppers are an excellent source of both vitamin C and carotenes, which help to neutralize the impact of harmful free radicals. Onions contain sulphur compounds, which may help to reduce blood pressure and ease inflammatory conditions, and they also have prebiotic properties that help to regulate levels of beneficial gut

THE RIGHT BITE

This is an excellent opportunity to choose a seafood option, as it will keep the calories and saturated fat content down, while allowing you to derive the benefit of healthy polyunsaturates. Choosing a skewer that has a generous range of vegetables interspersed with fish will transform it into a blood sugar-balancing option that supports optimal immune and digestive function.

bacteria. Cooking a tomato significantly increases levels of the antioxidant lycopene, which plays a key part in cardiovascular health as well as helping to reduce the risk of certain cancers.

AUBERGINE/EGGPLANT, PEPPERS AND TOMATOES are all members of the nightshade family. Individuals who are sensitive to these types of foods may experience a number of disparate symptoms, such as inflammation, joint pain, digestive difficulties, anxiety and headaches.

BAKED POTATO

A baked potato is commonly believed to be a healthy option and it's true that it's preferable to eating mashed potato, roast potato or fries. However, if your preference is to enjoy the fluffy potato in the middle and ignore the skin, you're doing yourself a disservice. The high-temperature baking process essentially breaks down the fibre of flesh, leaving a rapidly digestible carbohydrate that is likely to result in a blood sugar spike, leading to an energy dip and the munchies. By eating the skin, you'll increase your fibre intake and help to neutralize the rapid-release carbohydrate in the flesh, keeping you going for longer.

A CAREFUL CHOICE OF ACCOMPANIMENT with your baked potato can slow down the release of sugar into the bloodstream. Pairing it with some protein in the form of barbecued meat or fish, for example, makes this a nicely balanced dish that will help to keep extra inches at bay.

NUTRITION NUMBERS
per medium 200g potato (including skin)

↳ BAKED POTATO
Calories: 194 » Protein: 5g
Carbohydrate: 43g » Sugars: 3g
Fibre: 5g » Vitamin C: 12mg
Beta carotene: traces

↳ BAKED SWEET POTATO
Calories: 180 » Protein: 4g
Carbohydrate: 40g » Sugars: 13g
Fibre: 7g » Vitamin C: 34mg
Beta carotene: 7,920mcg

TOPPINGS

↳ BUTTER (per 25g serving)
Calories: 186 » Total fat: 20g
Saturated fat: 13g

↳ CHEDDAR CHEESE (per 50g serving)
Calories: 208 » Protein: 12g
Total fat: 17g » Saturated fat: 10g

The area just below the skin of any vegetable tends to be the richest in micronutrients and potatoes are no exception. Although not an important source of vitamins or minerals, they do contain some vitamin C and B vitamins, in particular vitamin B6, which plays a key role in the function of the nervous system. A deficiency in B6 may result in anxiety or depression.

Another option to consider is a baked sweet potato, which comes from quite a different family to the potato. Although the starch content appears roughly similar, and the sugar content even higher, they are widely considered to be a much better option when it comes to blood sugar management. Not only do they contain a generous dose of fibre, but sweet potatoes contain a protein hormone called adiponectin, which helps to regulate glucose levels in the body, an important consideration for anyone who is keen to avoid type 2 diabetes.

The other benefit of a sweet potato is the abundant antioxidants they contain, with extraordinarily high levels of beta carotene found in the orange flesh. A diet high in beta carotene and other antioxidants is believed to reduce the risk of some cancers by protecting against the activity of free radicals. Beta carotene also helps to promote eye health and improve night vision.

THE RIGHT BITE

If a baked sweet potato is on offer, then this is definitely the one to go for, as it has the dual benefit of supporting weight management and boosting immunity. If only standard potatoes are available, then it's best to opt for a smallish potato, so that you don't overdo the starch, and make sure you eat all the skin, to optimize fibre intake and help to neutralize the release of the starch in the body.

ADDING A SMALL AMOUNT OF FAT to a sweet potato can significantly increase the absorption of beta carotene. If you want to avoid using butter, a tablespoon of good-quality extra virgin olive oil can have just the same effect.

POTATO SALAD
& COLESLAW

A generous serving of potato salad can add up to a hefty calorie count as potatoes are extremely high in starch. Potato salad is commonly made with peeled potatoes and fibre levels are lower as a result; if you're making your own, use new potatoes in their skins, which will help to boost fibre content. Fibre helps to neutralize the release of the sugars generated by carbohydrate, keeping you going for longer.

Recent studies have shown that cold potatoes may have surprising health benefits, as the cooling process helps to create a more solid form of starch, known as resistant starch, which is not easily digested. Not only can this help to optimize digestive function, but it may

CABBAGE CONTAINS GLUCOSINOLATES, which studies have shown help to protect against a number of different cancers by reducing the growth of cancer cells.

NUTRITION NUMBERS
per 100g

↳ POTATO SALAD
Calories: 190 » Carbohydrate: 12g
Sugars: 2g » Fibre: 1g » Salt: 0.5g
Total fat: 14g » Saturated fat: 2g

↳ POTATO SALAD (low fat)
Calories: 107 » Carbohydrate: 12g
Sugars: 2g » Fibre: 1g » Salt: 0.5g
Total fat: 6g » Saturated fat: 0.5g

↳ COLESLAW
Calories: 219 » Carbohydrate: 5g
Sugars: 3g » Fibre: 2g » Salt: 0.5g
Total fat: 19g » Saturated fat: 2g

↳ COLESLAW (low fat)
Calories: 106 » Carbohydrate: 6g
Sugars: 5g » Fibre: 1g » Salt: 0.5g
Total fat: 9g » Saturated fat: 1g

also help to reduce the risk of colorectal cancers commonly associated with high levels of red meat.

Coleslaw is basically a mixture of grated cabbage and carrot, with occasional added onion, chives or peppers, according to regional variations. Whatever the blend, this is an excellent opportunity to boost your vegetable intake in a context that tends to be very meat and bread-heavy. Cabbage is the principal ingredient and is packed with antioxidant plant compounds such as polyphenols which help to reduce oxidative stress, a possible risk factor for cancer. Raw cabbage also helps to reduce cholesterol levels by facilitating the excretion of bile acids, although this is even more effective with lightly steamed cabbage.

The downside of these salads often comes with the dressings: with home-made versions, it's easier to control what you include. This can vary from home-made mayonnaise, to dressings containing buttermilk or white wine vinegar. The pitfalls tend to come with the commercial dressings that can be high in sugar and salt, especially a low-fat

THE RIGHT BITE

If it's an either/or situation, then full-fat coleslaw is the healthiest option. This adds a healthy portion of vegetables to your plate, increasing fibre intake for optimal digestion and exposing you to a range of protective antioxidants. If you generally prefer potato salad, then opting for a portion with full-fat dressing helps to ensure you avoid the additives and artificial flavourings commonly associated with low-fat versions.

dressing, as manufacturers often include additives and flavourings to compensate for the loss of flavour in a low-fat product.

FAT HELPS TO OPTIMISE THE ABSORPTION OF ANTIOXIDANTS in cabbage and carrots, such as carotenes and lycopene. Studies have shown that full-fat salad dressings enhance the absorption of antioxidants significantly more than low-fat dressings.

At the Movies

premiere choices

There's something about a trip to the movies that seems to send caution to the winds when it comes to snacking. Just a hint of the scent of popcorn or doughnuts as you walk through the doors seems to lead to an immediate diversion to the queue for the various outlets so you can stock up with goodies. As the lights go down, the rustling and crunching starts as everyone tucks into their snacks of choice.

Unfortunately there's little room for manoeuvre when it comes to keeping things healthy, unless you're prepared to smuggle some carrot sticks or a piece of fruit in with you. The biggest pitfall with movie snacks tends to be the high levels of sugar and refined carbohydrate, so if you still want to indulge, the trick is to keep the portions small and limit the sugary toppings or glazings. If you're not a natural sharer and hate the idea of someone else picking at your food, the moviehouse is one place where you might want to bend the rules, as this can make a big difference to just how much you actually consume.

> The trick is to keep the portions small and limit the sugary toppings or glazes

Opting for a savoury snack in a bid to keep sugar levels down may seem like a smart move, but beware of exposing yourself to the excessive levels of saturated fat and trans fats, as these are commonly found in processed meats. However, a clever selection of toppings for nachos can provide some surprising health benefits, including regulation of cholesterol levels, reduced risk of cardiovascular disease and protective antioxidants.

All in all, going to the movies can be a bit of a health minefield, but as in so many cases, moderation is the key, so if you're only indulging in one of these treats every few months, then it's unlikely to be an issue. However, regular movie-goers should take note, as there is a price to pay for tucking into these foods on a weekly (or more regular) basis.

POPCORN

Popcorn is derived from the kernel of maize that expands and puffs up when exposed to heat. As the heat builds, the pressure on the kernel increases, which is what leads to the popping sound when preparing it.

It's commonly considered to be a healthy snack and while it is extremely high in starch, in its basic form it offers a wholegrain snack with a decent amount of fibre that is likely to promote sustained energy levels far longer than other popular snacks. Research has shown that snacking on small amounts of popcorn compared to potato chips

TUCKING INTO A LARGE PORTION OF SALTED POPCORN means that you'll be having two-thirds of the recommended daily limit of 6g of salt. If blood pressure is a concern, this is one to avoid, as it's likely to leave you well over the limit, once you've taken into account everything else you've eaten during the day.

NUTRITION NUMBERS

↳ SWEET POPCORN (small)
Calories: 473 » Protein: 6g
Carbohydrate: 57g » Sugars: 17g
Fibre: 9g » Fat: 15g » Salt: 0.02g

↳ SWEET POPCORN (large)
Calories: 985 » Protein: 13g
Carbohydrate: 120g » Sugars: 36g
Fibre: 19g » Fat: 41g » Salt: 0.06g

↳ SALTED POPCORN (small)
Calories: 432 » Protein: 7g
Carbohydrate: 47g » Sugars: 0.6g
Fibre: 11g » Fat: 20g » Salt: 1.6g

↳ SALTED POPCORN (large)
Calories: 910 » Protein: 14g
Carbohydrate: 90g » Sugars: 1.2g
Fibre: 23g » Fat: 37g » Salt: 4g

enhances satiety, which may make it a preferred option for people who want to reduce feelings of hunger and increase energy levels.

However, the reality is that almost no one snacks on popcorn in its basic form and the offerings available for snacking at the movies have generous additions of butter, sugar, caramel and salt, depending on your choice. In all cases this is transforming a potentially healthy snack into something that is going to have an immediate impact on your waistline. Depending on the choice of portion, you could be consuming the equivalent of anything between 4 and 9 teaspoons of sugar, without even taking into account the starchy carbohydrate in the snack.

A further challenge is the fact that portion size appears to go out of the window when we hit the movies and as the lights go down so does all sense of proportion as we tuck into giant buckets of popcorn, consuming quantities that would be unthinkable in a more mindful eating situation. There's little to choose between the calories in a large portion of sweet or salted popcorn: either way it's going to add up to about half the daily

THE RIGHT BITE

If weight management is your goal, then it's really best to avoid popcorn altogether. However, sharing a small portion between two or three people can help to limit the damage and by opting for savoury rather than sweet popcorn, sugar levels will be kept to a minimum.

recommended amount of calories for women.

While it's true that salted popcorn contains considerably less sugar than sweetened forms, this is no reason to overindulge, as the high carbohydrate content still makes this a starchy snack, which the body will break down into sugar almost immediately.

THE HULLS OF POPCORN (that commonly get caught in the teeth) are a concentrated source of beneficial polyphenols, considered to have protective antioxidant properties.

ICE CREAM

The basic ingredients of traditional ice cream are milk, cream and sugar with some form of flavouring or fruit, so it's not surprising that this most indulgent of treats is so high in calories. This combination of fat and sugar is the ultimate comfort food and while excessive consumption of sugar is the single biggest factor when it comes to gaining inches, current thinking suggests that regularly eating foods that are both high in fat and sugar is incredibly addictive to our taste buds and can result in steady weight gain.

In recent years, more and more complex flavours and blends of ice cream have become available and with that, levels of sugar (as well as additives and flavourings) have increased exponentially,

SOME CHEAPER BRANDS OF ICE CREAM may contain fat in the form of hydrogenated vegetable fats, otherwise known as trans fats, which can impact cholesterol levels and result in fatty deposits in the arteries.

NUTRITION NUMBERS
per 2 scoops (170g)

↳ VANILLA ICE CREAM
Calories: 332 » Carbohydrate: 33g
Sugars: 26g » Saturated fat: 13g

↳ CHOCOLATE/CARAMEL ICE CREAM
Calories: 369 » Carbohydrate: 43g
Sugars: 34g » Saturated fat: 16g

↳ CHOC-CHIP COOKIE ICE CREAM
Calories: 383 » Carbohydrate: 31g
Sugars: 28g » Saturated fat: 18g

↳ STRAWBERRY CHEESECAKE ICE CREAM
Calories: 382 » Carbohydrate: 38g
Sugars: 32g » Saturated fat: 13g

↳ NATURAL FROZEN YOGURT (100g pot)
Calories: 150 » Carbohydrate: 38g
Sugars: 26g » Saturated fat: 3g

↳ PASSION FRUIT FROZEN YOGURT (100g pot)
Calories: 160 » Carbohydrate: 36g
Sugars: 28g » Saturated fat: 3g

with even a modest serving of ice cream containing 7–8 teaspoons of sugar. A helping of chocolate or caramel sauce adds over 300 calories, so the whole treat can be more than a quarter of the recommended daily calorie intake for women in just one small serving.

Despite the name, many ice creams may often contain surprisingly low levels of milk and cream and it is becoming increasingly common for vegetable oils to feature in ice cream as a fat replacement. Although levels of dairy produce are regulated in order for a product to qualify as ice cream, in the UK, for example, ice cream only needs to contain 2.5% milk protein and 5% milk fat to fulfil the requirements. Ice cream which is labelled as 'dairy', however, cannot contain any other form of fat, so it's worth paying attention to the label.

Frozen yogurt has become increasingly popular in recent years and is hailed as the low-fat, low-calorie healthy alternative to ice cream. However, a quick glance at the numbers reveals that all is not what it seems. It's lower in fat than a standard ice cream, but the sugar levels tend to be roughly the same

THE RIGHT BITE

It's best to keep things simple with ice cream or frozen yogurt – while it's never going to be a low-sugar option, you can limit the damage by opting for just a small portion and a simple flavour, such as vanilla, avoiding any sugary toppings. Ideally aim for a product labelled as dairy, so that you can be sure that you're limiting your potential exposure to trans fats.

as so much is added in the way of sugary flavours. If weight loss is your goal, frozen yogurt is unlikely to be much kinder to your waistline than a tub of ice cream.

BE WARY OF CLAIMS THAT FROZEN YOGURT contains 'probiotic' bacteria that can support digestive health. Levels are likely to vary dramatically depending on the product and in any case the levels tend to be low to insignificant. It might be considered a potential small advantage but shouldn't be the main reason for consuming the product.

DOUGHNUTS

Creating a mixture of sugar, butter, eggs and flour and then deep-frying it and rolling it in sugar, icing it or injecting it with cream or jam is never going to produce the healthiest of snacks. If you're a doughnut fan, you need to be aware that there is very little to recommend them in nutrition terms and in fact much damage can be done if you overindulge.

The blend of sugar and fat found in doughnuts is an artificial combination that doesn't exist in nature and research suggests that it can disrupt the satiety mechanisms in the body. The result is that such an addictive blend is likely to leave you craving more in the way of this type of comfort food, which will have a hugely negative impact on your waistline.

RESEARCH HAS SHOWN that eating deep-fried carbohydrate products such as doughnuts more than once a week may be associated with an increased risk of contracting prostate cancer.

NUTRITION NUMBERS
per unit

↳ CHOCOLATE ICED RING DOUGHNUT

Calories: 250 » Carbohydrate: 32g
Sugars: 21g » Fat: 21g

↳ GLAZED RING DOUGHNUT

Calories: 206 » Carbohydrate: 22g
Sugars: 15g » Fat: 13g

↳ JAM-FILLED DOUGHNUT

Calories: 320 » Carbohydrate: 37g
Sugars: 18g » Fat: 16g

↳ CHOCOLATE CUSTARD-FILLED DOUGHNUT

Calories: 360 » Carbohydrate: 35g
Sugars: 20g » Fat: 22g

The sugar levels of doughnuts are a particular concern. Popular flavoured doughnuts that come with chocolate icing or chocolate fudge, for example, contain 6–8 teaspoons of sugar, and that's without counting the refined carbohydrate that the body will break down into sugar almost immediately. There is no getting past the fact that a doughnut is basically a big ball of sugar.

It's not just about the ingredients, however, because the cooking method also plays a key part in the health impact of doughnuts and the dangers of frying food at very high temperatures are well documented. Artificial trans fats are formed when manufacturers add hydrogen to unsaturated fats to increase the shelf life of products and the melting point of the fat, which allows for cooking at very high temperatures. While the jury might be out on saturated fat, there is no dispute about the connection between trans fats and the impact on cholesterol levels and the risk of heart disease.

The move to legislate against the use of trans fats in the USA has led some popular doughnut chains to exclude them, but do you know if your favourite doughnut contains them? In any case, even if the trans fats are removed, frying at high temperatures has been linked to an increased risk of some cancers, so doughnuts need to be treated with caution.

THE RIGHT BITE

Ideally, you would choose a different snack but if you're desperate for a doughnut, then the least damage is likely to be done by opting for a simple glazed version. You won't be able to avoid the issues linked to eating deep-fried food, but the sugar content is roughly half of what you'll find in a more elaborate doughnut.

HIGH LEVELS OF SUGAR can have a detrimental effect on digestion by encouraging an overgrowth of unfriendly bacteria in the gut, leading to bloating, wind and digestive discomfort. If you struggle in this area, it may be time to cut back on eating sugary doughnuts.

HOT DOG

Traditionally a frankfurter sausage in a long bun, the hot dog has been a staple snack in some countries for centuries. However, modern processing methods and the requirement to keep costs to a minimum have brought a whole new dimension to the traditional frankfurter, which has resulted in a highly processed product that has some very real health implications. This means that the average commercial hot dog should be treated with caution.

As with all meat-based products, it all comes down to the quality of the meat itself. Hot dogs are commonly made with

HELPING YOURSELF TO A GENEROUS PORTION OF MUSTARD could be a good idea. Traditionally held to have a number of medicinal qualities, mustard contains anti-inflammatory compounds and is a good source of selenium, an antioxidant that is believed to help protect against some cancers.

NUTRITION NUMBERS

↳ PORK FRANKFURTER (regular)
Calories: 184 » Protein: 10g
Carbohydrate: 3g » Sugars: 0.8g
Total fat: 15g » Saturated fat: 6g
Salt: 1.5g

↳ PORK FRANKFURTER (large)
Calories: 293 » Protein: 13g
Carbohydrate: 5g » Sugars: 1g
Total fat: 26g » Saturated fat: 10g
Salt: 2.6g

↳ TOTAL HOT DOG (regular, including bun)
Calories: 415 » Protein: 18g
Carbohydrate: 50g » Sugars: 7g
Total fat: 20g » Saturated fat: 7g
Salt: 2.5g

↳ TOTAL HOT DOG (large, including bun)
Calories: 524 » Protein: 21g
Carbohydrate: 52g » Sugars: 7g
Total fat: 31g » Saturated fat: 11g
Salt: 3.6g

pork trimmings (this is what's left after the bacon, ham and chops have been cut out) and then mixed with poultry. In some cases, where costs are kept to a minimum, mechanically separated meat can be used and this is where a machine blasts off the remaining meat from a butchered carcass creating a type of meat paste.

The meat mixture is blended with water, starch, flavourings and additives, inserted into a plastic tube for cooking and then packaged up for commercial use. One of the key additives that is commonly included is sodium nitrite, which is used to preserve the pink colour of processed meats, even after cooking. Excessive consumption of processed meats has been associated with the increased risk of some cancers and some research suggests that nitrates may be a contributory factor.

Beware of the bun, as it's usually highly processed and contains almost 250 calories on its own, as well as a generous dose of sugar, which makes the bread sweeter and more addictive.

Hot dogs are a high salt food – just one hot dog can exceed the

THE RIGHT BITE

It's very difficult to find an upside with hot dogs, as they are a highly processed product. Ideally, they should be avoided, but if you do enjoy the occasional treat, then make sure it's just that – i.e. something that you only eat every few months, rather than tucking in once a week.

daily recommended limit of salt for young children, and is easily half the amount recommended for adults. This is definitely a snack to be wary of on a family outing, as excessive levels of salt can contribute to high blood pressure and may increase the risk of cardiovascular disease.

ALL SAUSAGES (even quality organic offerings) contain some form of starch as a binder. With hot dogs this is commonly potato starch or rusk, which is mixed with the meat paste and water to create the soft texture associated with the frankfurter.

NACHOS

Tortilla chips are a hugely popular snack, especially when served in the form of nachos with all the associated toppings and dips. Although they're made from corn rather than potatoes, the nutritional breakdown is very similar to potato chips, in that they're a very carb-heavy, salted snack which is deep-fried in vegetable oil. A regular 100g serving of just plain tortilla chips adds up to over 500 calories and if you enjoy some sugary drinks or beer at the same time, then you can easily double this in a very short space of time.

Nachos themselves are available with a variety of toppings and by making a

TOMATO SALSA IS A LOW-FAT OPTION that doesn't just taste great but has the added advantage of being a rich source of the antioxidant lycopene. Recent research has shown that lycopene can help to reduce the risk of heart disease. It's also believed to be important for male health as it may help to reduce the risk of prostate cancer.

NUTRITION NUMBERS
per 100g serving

↳ **NACHOS WITH MELTED CHEESE (regular)**
Calories: 658 » Carbohydrate: 68g
Total fat: 28g » Saturated fat: 6g
Protein: 8g » Fibre: 8g

↳ **GUACAMOLE (per 30g serving)**
Calories: 50 » Carbohydrate: 2g
Total fat: 5g » Saturated fat: 1g
Protein: 1g » Fibre: 1g

↳ **TOMATO SALSA (per 30g serving)**
Calories: 15 » Carbohydrate: 4.5g
Fibre: 1g

↳ **SOUR CREAM (per 30g serving)**
Calories: 68 » Carbohydrate: 1g
Total fat: 7g » Saturated fat: 4g
Protein: 1g

↳ **BEANS (per 30g serving)**
Calories: 100 » Carbohydrate: 18g
Total fat: 1g » Saturated fat: 0.3g
Protein: 7g » Fibre: 7g

smart choice, it's possible to turn them into a satisfying snack that is likely to keep you going for longer and reduce the chances of reaching for another snack an hour or so later. The trick here is to be generous with the beans and the guacamole, as it significantly boosts the protein and fibre content. This will help neutralize the impact of the high carbohydrate content of the snack and help your body to produce sustained energy, rather than a quick burst of energy that leaves you needing another carb boost in a short space of time.

A large serving of melted cheese is never going to be the healthiest choice, but if you can steer yourself away from that and toward the guacamole, re-fried beans and tomato salsa, then you're picking a more sustaining option that contains some residual health benefits that may surprise you. Avocado, found in guacamole, is a rich source of monounsaturated fats that can help to regulate cholesterol levels and it also contains potassium, which plays a key role in heart health.

Pinto beans are a 5-star source of nutrients with a range of health benefits.

THE RIGHT BITE

The smart move here is to keep the cheese and the sour cream to a minimum and tuck into the guacamole, salsa and beans. If you can eat more of the topping and less of the tortilla chips, this will also help to keep the calorie content down.

As well as being an excellent source of protein and fibre to stabilize blood sugar levels, reduce sugar cravings and provide sustained energy, regular consumption of beans is believed to reduce the risk of a heart attack. Pinto beans are also rich in detoxifying molybdenum and energy-rich iron as well as protective antioxidants.

IF YOU'RE A FAN OF SPICY FOOD, then it's a good idea to get an extra helping of jalapeño onto your nachos. Chilli peppers are packed with antioxidants and plant compounds known as flavonoids, which are believed to have a protective effect against some cancers.

INDEX

ABOUT THE AUTHOR

Jackie Lynch is a Registered Nutritional Therapist and the founder of the WellWellWell nutritional therapy clinic in West London. Passionate about the importance of good food for optimum health, Jackie focuses on providing practical advice that helps support a busy 21st-century lifestyle and is a sought-after speaker for nutrition talks and workshops. With her accessible approach to making good food choices, Jackie's advice features in a wide range of national publications and she has appeared as a guest expert on television and radio lifestyle programmes. Visit her website at: www.well-well-well.co.uk.

ACKNOWLEDGEMENTS

Special thanks are due to all the team at Nourish, in particular James Spackman and Grace Cheetham for commissioning the concept; editors Elinor Brett, Rebecca Woods and Dawn Bates, for their sterling work; designer Viki Ottewill for making it look so beautiful; and the publicity and rights teams for all their help. My friends have shown unfailing enthusiasm for this project and, for this, I thank you all. None of this would have been possible without the support of all my lovely family, especially my late mother Terry, to whom this book is dedicated; my father Frank, for teaching me that anything is possible; my sister Frankie, for her daily advice and encouragement; and my brother Rob, a constant source of ideas and inspiration.

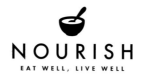

NOURISH
EAT WELL, LIVE WELL

Here at Nourish we're all about wellbeing through food and drink – irresistible dishes with a serious good-for-you factor. If you want to eat and drink delicious things that set you up for the day, suit any special diets, keep you healthy and make the most of the ingredients you have, we've got some great ideas to share with you. Come over to our blog for wholesome recipes and fresh inspiration – nourishbooks.com